IT'S
AN INSIDE JOB!

EMOTIONAL HEALTH
SECRETS
OF A
LYMPHOMANIAC

♥

JUDY HINEY TAYLOR

IT'S AN INSIDE JOB!
EMOTIONAL HEALTH SECRETS
OF A LYMPHOMANIAC

by Judy Hiney Taylor

With Foreword by Dr. Patricia Fitzgerald, Founder, The Santa Monica Wellness Center

Life Source Productions, Santa Monica, CA 90403

Published in 2006

Printed in Morrisville, N.C.

ISBN 978-0-6151-3678-3

Emotional intelligence is a different way of being smart.
It includes knowing your feelings and using them to make good decisions;
managing your feelings well; motivating yourself with zeal and persistence;
maintaining hope in the face of frustration; exhibiting empathy and compassion;
interacting smoothly; and managing your relationships effectively.
Those emotional skills matter immensely...

Daniel Goleman,
author of *Emotional Intelligence*

♥

*Our mental and emotional diets determine
our overall energy levels, health, and well-being
to a far greater extent than most people realize.*

Doc Childre and Howard Martin,
authors of *The HeartMath Solution*

♥

DEDICATION

To my dear mother,
whose last words were
"Please finish your book!"
and to my family,
my greatest blessing!

♥

*Health and peace in the world
begin inside each one of us.*

It's an Inside Job!

♥

Contents

Contents - continued

Contents - continued

Lymphomaniac: *Someone who is crazy in love with the healing powers of the Lymphatic System. Though largely unknown, the Lymphatic System is a crucial partner to the Immune System, and it also cleanses and detoxifies the body through its massive network of organs and vessels. For over 18 years, the author has been documenting the connection that the lymphatic system has with our emotions. To learn more about the lymph, turn ahead to the Lymphatic System section.*

Wisdom begins with wonder.

Socrates

♥

Foreword

Ask people today what their stress level is, and the answer is often "very high" or "I am always stressed." We live in a fast-paced society where feeling overwhelmed and out of balance is common. Now we're witnessing this phenomenon taking its toll on our health.

Continual research mounts to verify the stress-disease connection. In my own practice, I have experienced thousands of clients who have told me *unsolicited* that they believed their illness was the result of stress. What's the answer? I think it's time to look at *how we respond emotionally* to the stress in our lives.

It's an Inside Job! is a wonderful culmination of Judy Taylor's clinical experience in the holistic health field. Ms. Taylor wrote her book after realizing how crucial emotional healing and emotional wisdom are to our well-being. As a healthcare practitioner for over twenty years myself, I can passionately applaud Ms. Taylor's emphasis. Whenever I take a history of a new client who has a chronic illness, and I ask if there was a history of chronic emotional stress in childhood or a stress pattern around the time of the onset of the illness, the answer is virtually always "yes."

Fortunately, Chinese medical theory has always viewed emotional and physical health as integrated, so it has been a natural progression for me as a practitioner of Traditional Chinese Medicine to work on various levels to facilitate healing in my clients. My colleagues and I are truly blessed to continually witness mind-body-spirit healing. In fact, traditional natural medical systems throughout the world emphasize emotional healing as crucial to any healing process.

An awareness is growing among mainstream American medicine of the importance of stress and the emotional component. Yet most medical personnel will acknowledge that they are often not equipped to teach clients stress management or emotional health strategies. Interestingly, most medical personnel could probably use these techniques for their own benefit. So I welcome the entrance of Judy Taylor as an author who is contributing to the dialogue of what is important for our well-being.

When I think of Judy Taylor and her book, two common phrases come to mind... "Practice what you preach" and "Experience is everything." When you're looking for guidance in a particular area, it is wise to find a teacher who walks the talk. By this I mean, they provide inspiration, not just information. Judy Taylor does that. A cancer survivor, she has spent decades improving her own state of wellness, and Ms. Taylor shares the lessons she has lived in this book.

But the lessons are not only from Ms. Taylor's own life. What is extraordinary here is to be able to gain wisdom on how to embody these ideas from someone who has had (literally) hands on experience of witnessing and facilitating the emotional health improvements of real people. By facilitating lymphatic therapy, Ms. Taylor has been an integral part of the increased well-being of many grateful people.

Socrates once said, "Wisdom begins with wonder." Wonder involves looking at life as a journey of learning, growing, and loving. Judy Taylor is a woman who has lived well and can therefore offer us her timeless wisdom and insights so we can soar to new heights. Who of us is wise enough to accept the challenge?

Dr. Patricia Fitzgerald, L.Ac., C.C.N., D.H.M.
Author, *The Detox Solution*
Founder, The Santa Monica Wellness Center, Santa Monica, CA

*This book is offered as
both a guide and a resource
to encourage transformations
for a healthier and more balanced life.*

♥

Introduction

Why would a Lymphomaniac write a book about emotional health? To begin to explain, I need to go back to the early years of my life.

As a young girl, I fell in love with the mind and our emotions. I was optimistic and enormously curious as to why each person was different and about what attracted me to some people much more than others. I even asked my parents if I could go to therapy to see what made people "tick." Issues with my dad (which ultimately made me a better person) were another reason I wanted to go to see a psychiatrist.

Guess what? Soon my parents supported my request and there I was in therapy! But what I didn't know was that I'd do all the talking and the psychiatrist, who I wanted to communicate with me, would just sit there and wait for me to talk some more. When I asked him, "Please tell me about yourself," he refused. Well, so much for therapy! I stopped going. However, kids recognize their truth. I think I must have wanted to be in a profession that works with the emotions even back then.

In fact, my interest and curiosity about the mind and our emotions never left me. I kept studying psychology over the years. And then who would have thought that opening up a health spa during my forties in Ojai, California would have led me to becoming a Lymphomaniac and realizing my dream job?

Here's how it happened. By suggestion from a chiropractor, I became a Lymphatic Therapist and added lymphatic massage to our services at the spa. Very quickly, I became impressed by the lymph system. But can you guess what the main reason was that I became a Lymphomaniac?... Yes? No? Well, I saw that lymphatic therapy was not only a remarkable way to cleanse and detoxify the body, but also the mind and our emotions. And I found that issues with the mind and our emotions are the root cause of *most issues* with health!

What else did I see? I saw that the body holds onto emotional information related to thoughts we hold in our minds. And each part of the body represents a different part of the mind. So there it was – my opportunity to work on the physical body where the emotional blockages were and deal with the mental and emotional issues that had fascinated me all of my life! When I worked on the blocked areas of the lymph system, the lumps, bumps, swelling or pain disappeared. And clients found that they were then able to get in touch with difficult emotions and thoughts that they were holding onto, and release them.

For instance, one client found that after her first visit, her emotional body opened up again, after many years of being shut down. After her second visit, she experienced the feeling of fear surfacing in her life and began to work through it. After her third visit, she remembered times when she saw physical violence. Then with some more lymphatic work, she was able to release the trauma associated with these memories – a move she feels was life-changing! By clearing her Lymphatic System, she was also clearing her energetic core of emotional residue from the past.

So now you understand how I gained knowledge about emotional health and became a Lymphomaniac. But why did I write this book? Well, you see, every day your emotional health impacts your physical well-being in dynamic ways. (More on this in "The Mind-Body Connection" section, which is coming up ahead.) In particular, it enables your lymph system to do a better job in its important role as a cleanser, detoxifier and immunity builder. Therefore, to help you gain mastery of your emotions and your thoughts, I'm sharing the wisdom I have gained and emotional health secrets I have learned. The chapters in my book will explore aspects of life that you experience daily.

I am honored to share my experiences, my knowledge and my heart with you. This book is offered as both a guide and a resource to encourage transformations for a healthier and more balanced life. It provides information, reflection and solace for those who want to understand the mysteries of the inner self and deepen their experience of it. And your healing will be important for the healing of the planet.

Health and peace in the world begin inside each one of us. *It's an Inside Job!*

The Lymphatic System:

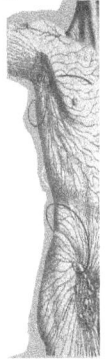

A Largely Unknown,
But Dynamic Health Partner

Did you know?...

Our Lymphatic System consists of a complex set of organs and vessels, designed to ward off infection, germs, and disease. It works in concert with our immune system.

The Lymphatic System channels its way throughout the body, carrying infection-fighting cells, and filtering impurities. It is commonly known as the "garbage disposal system" of the body.

♥ The Lymphatic System is crucial to the cleansing of the body!

♥ It destroys harmful bacteria, fungi, and other toxic materials!

♥ The Lymphatic System has no pump and relies on the body's exercise and breath to function optimally!

♥ A Healthy Nervous System depends on a Healthy Lymph System!

♥ You have four times more lymph fluid than you have blood!

My findings over the past 18 years regarding the connection between the workings of the lymph system and emotional well-being led to the writing of this book *It's an Inside Job! Emotional Health Secrets of a Lymphomaniac.*

A merry heart
makes good medicine.

The Book of Proverbs

♥

The Mind-Body Connection

Should the body be treated separately from the mind and our emotions? There's a truth that I have personally experienced through my own self-healing from cancer and in observations of my clients – *the body and mind work together.*

But you don't have to trust just my personal observations. There's been plenty of research which validates the mind-body connection. In particular, I am attracted to the work of Candace Pert. In her book *Molecules of Emotion*, this internationally recognized researcher writes, "Most psychologists treat the mind as disembodied, a phenomenon with little or no connection to the physical body. Conversely physicians treat the body with no regard to the mind or the emotions. But the body and mind are not separate..."

A pharmacologist, Pert found that the vital link between body and mind is *in the emotions and their biological components.* Dr. Pert believes that the emotions coordinate all parts of our physiology into one harmonious whole. In her ground-breaking book *Molecules of Emotion*, this author explains that the "chemistry of emotion" is what allows the mind and body to communicate. And she tells us that emotions can be found in our muscles, organs, glands, brain and stomach (talk about "gut feelings"!). In fact, one of her most stunning discoveries is that emotional information is held in the body at a *cellular level.*

More commonly known mind-body research has linked psychological and emotional stress to high blood pressure, chest pain, heart attacks, and even death. For instance, a study of clients with coronary heart disease by Dr. Diwaker Jain of the Yale Medical School appeared in *The Journal of the American College of Cardiology* (May 1998). His conclusion? *Mental stress is at least as potent as physical stress in the exacerbation of heart disease.*

In watching my own healing and that of others, I have seen that lightening up, loving and laughing can be more healing than any drug out on the market. And in his book, *The Healing Diet: A Total Health Program to Purify Your Lymph System and Reduce the Risk of Heart Disease*, cardiologist Gerald M. Lemole, M.D. echoes my view about the power of laughter and a light heart with the comment: "It delights me to think that Robin Williams or Richard Pryor have had a greater impact on the nation's health than any other number of gray-faced doctors prescribing Xanax or Percocet." He adds that the benefit of laughter comes in part from the resulting change in our physiological environment – one of relaxation and calmness.

And what feels better than to be touched... emotionally or physically? An early pioneer in mind/body interactions, Ilana Rubenfeld has explored the psychological benefits of touch through her Rubenfeld Synergy Method. This system for emotional healing combines compassionate bodywork with Gestalt therapy and intuition. Backed by over 40 years of research, Rubenfeld's findings prove that memories and emotions stored in our bodies can result in blocked energy and imbalances. Her book *The Listening Hand* describes how to use her method for self-healing.

In my own practice as a lymphatic specialist, I utilize a special bodywork technique, which was pioneered by the Danish therapists Emil and Estrid Vodder in the 1930s. Called Manual Lymphatic Drainage (MLD), it is a way of gently palpating and moving the skin to stimulate the circulation of the lymph. It can be used for many ailments, helping to relieve swelling, bruising, lumps, bumps and pain – all of which are signs of lymphatic blockage. Though I originally learned the technique to help people with physical challenges, I found a cleansing of the mind and emotions to be effected as well. (You'll find further details on this in the Introduction.) Once again, we see the mind-body link.

Yes, the mind, body and emotions are integrated and inseparable! It is an energy system which maintains our health. The key to staying healthy then is to care for the whole body through *balance*. Bring balance out of the chaos in your life! I know you can do it! And we'll start with emotional balance... with this book leading the way.

Have enough trust, honor and faith
in your own self
to acknowledge, express
and live your truth.

♥

The Emotional You And The Power You Have

To be healthy and happy, feeling vibrant and very much alive... you have the power to make it all happen! By gaining greater emotional mastery, and better self-understanding, you will be loving yourself. And then your lymph will be better able to support you in becoming the person you always wanted to be. My book will get you started down this path.

What's the answer to keeping the lymphatics and your life flowing? Having enough trust, honor, and faith in your own self to acknowledge, express and live your truth. Be who you are, always with kindness and gentleness. This will support your lymphatic system, which in turn will keep your immune system in tiptop shape. It will also help you achieve a balanced life.

Keep reading to learn how to honor yourself, your emotions, and your health more each day!

Now that you know
honoring yourself is the ticket,
why not tune into a station
called YOU?

♥

1 Letting Your Emotions Guide You

The emotions inside you are a good guide to consult regarding how to care for your body, mind, and spirit. When you acknowledge yourself by choosing to listen *to you*, this creates positive movement in life. And doesn't it make sense that when you're in tune to yourself, your lymphatic system will be positively affected?

Now that you know that honoring yourself is the ticket, why not tune into a station called *YOU*? By doing so, you will be doing away with resistance and keeping yourself alive in a powerful way. So remember to embrace your feelings and then follow their lead – which is *your lead* – for guidance.

A great process is to make a list of the ideas for guidance that come to you, plus how you act on them. Do this for a week or so, and see what the results are. By monitoring your reality and becoming aware of whether you are following your inside prompt, you'll be able to assess the gifts you enjoyed or ignored. If you didn't act on your inner wisdom, ask yourself, "Why not?" See if you can do better the next time. And when you do follow up your inner wisdom with action, give yourself acknowledgement for facing the things you need to work on in your life! Then go have some fun!

You see, your emotions are your reflection of where you are in life... and you take them with you wherever you go. Sometimes we're flying high with joy, knowing we're on track with our life; other times, we're wading through difficult emotions, which give us the message to make changes.

But, eventually, honoring your own truth shall set you free! You'll spend less time wading through the muck. And the highs you'll experience from being emotionally free are like flying as a kite way up in a bright open sky!

So how are you programming your life and your lymphatic health? A good beginning is knowing that your lymph system listens to you!!! However, how well are you listening to yourself?

♥ **A point to consider:** Listening to myself positively affects my life and my lymphatic system.

♥ **Affirmation:** My interior guide is there for my greater good.

♥ **A question to ask:** Why wouldn't I listen to my own guidance?

If you keep focusing on the drama,
don't be surprised when your life becomes
that drama even more.

♥

2 Paying Too Much Attention To Our Drama And Trauma

I love what American author Henry Miller had to say:

"Develop interest in life as you see it; in people, things, literature, music – the world is so rich. Simply throbbing with rich treasures, beautiful souls, and interesting people. FORGET YOURSELF."

You need not pay too much attention to your drama and trauma. You need to pay more attention to gratitude and life's many possibilities. Life was designed for our enjoyment, not to be experienced as an endurance test!

Now, don't get me wrong; there are times when we're given circumstances that definitely bring up tender feelings – emotions that are rocky and throw us off balance for a bit. But at these times, you can slow down and ask yourself:

- ♥ "What's the good that I can see from this?"

- ♥ "What's the message that I need to get out of this?"

- ♥ "What will this circumstance make me remember and how can it affect me for the better?"

It's quite amazing when you think about it; you could easily become your drama and stories. So if you keep focusing on the drama, don't be surprised when your life becomes that drama even more, and if this continues for as long as you hold onto your stories.

Doesn't it sound better to experience the feelings, acknowledge the reality, and trust that you're allowed to move onto a new place – a better place! It's called... *get a life!*

♥ **A point to consider:** Drama and trauma create more drama and trauma.

♥ **Affirmation:** I am allowed to experience my feelings, and then move on.

♥ **A question to ask:** What is it that I need? Why am I staying in my drama and trauma?

Do you give yourself
support, honor, and respect?

♥

3   Your #1 Relationship – The One With Yourself

It is quite a gift to have relationships. They come in every shape and form, and are always being created every step of the way. Just think about it. For instance, there is your relationship with yourself #1. That is the biggie! It's what forms the foundation for all the other relationships in your life.

Please stop for a moment. Close your eyes and picture what your #1 relationship feels like to you. How it feels to you is exactly how it feels to your lymphatic system. And it is that reflection which shows up in your health and sense of well-being. This feeling is also the foundation for your total being out in the world and in your world... and it comes from the inside out.

Do you give yourself support, honor, and respect? Do you listen to that voice inside saying that because you are you, you are entitled to express all of what that is... all of whatever it is that defines your own uniqueness? After all, if everyone was meant to be the same in life, we would have been designed to look the same, have the same desires, exhibit the same talents, and share the same likes and dislikes. Does that sound like a very interesting world? No way! In fact, it is loving, liking, and appreciating the differences in each of us that creates a good relationship with yourself and other people.

Is your heart open when you make decisions? Do you see yourself as a worthy person? Do you feel you deserve to be treated lovingly? Can you give love and receive it too? If the answers to these questions are yes, you are most likely having a good relationship with yourself. If the answer is no to any of these questions, it is a good idea to allow yourself a better life. And a healthier lymphatic system. Let go of the judgments and blame of yourself and others! No one gave us the right to be judgmental.

You create the circumstances and relationships that either support you or not, and your choices affect your lymphatic system. So be good to yourself. There is only one person designed to be all that you are. It is right to give love to yourself. *You are special.*

The relationship you have with yourself creates the template for all the relationships you encounter in all of your life – be it intimacy, work, friendship, family and even momentary encounters like with a checker at the supermarket. Give yourself the gift of enjoying your natural right to have loving relationships as you go through this wonderful thing called life. Your lymph system will be grateful and supportive when you do.

- ♥ **A point to consider:** My relationship with myself creates the template for all of my relationships.
- ♥ **Affirmation:** I can have good relationships by having a good relationship with myself.
- ♥ **A question to ask:** When I look at my relationships, do I see that I am or am not experiencing love?

*There's no end to
the delights of life
you could enjoy
if only you'd notice them.*

♥

4 Experiencing Delight

The truth of a life really has little to do with what happens. Does that surprise you? The quality of your life is actually derived from your ability to experience DELIGHT. And the openness for DELIGHT comes from the gift of paying attention – from looking and listening, by being in the moment. When you pay attention to your world's delights, your lymphatic healing can take place.

Just think of how many things there are in the world that touch you, that make you feel good, that bring you joy – perhaps even tears of joy! *Is it the smile of someone walking towards you – a friendly stranger or someone you know? Is it simply taking in the beauty and scent of a flower, enjoying the sensational blue sky with its clouds delicately floating by, and oh so many other wonderful creations of Mother Nature? Is it a baby kicking its darling little feet and waving its precious hands for no reason?* There's no end to the delights of life you could enjoy if only you'd notice them. If you don't choose to notice – then and only then are there no delights!

Since we have free will as human beings, we have a choice whether to experience delight or not. *We choose to* or not. But remember that the lymphatic system is affected by our emotions and expressions. Why not support both your life and your health by appreciating the delights that this wonderful world has to offer?

When you change your focus to delight, your sense of awareness will fill up with so much positive energy! This will help balance the times when you are given uncomfortable circumstances and opportunities to catapult you to a new and better place in your life. Delight will be the thing that lifts you up!

- ♥ **A point to consider:** I have a choice to experience the delights of life.

- ♥ **Affirmation:** Life is worth delighting in.

- ♥ **A question to ask:** How would life be different for me if I delighted in the many opportunities that come my way?

Our Inner Critic beats us up
for having lives
that don't seem to be
working for us.

♥

5 Letting Go Of Your Internal Critic

Close your eyes, become still, and get in touch with your inner self. This is a way to receive answers regarding the situations that cause you to be so hard on yourself. When you are silent and listening to yourself, you also have the opportunity to get rid of your Inner Critic. The Critic is the internal part of you that puts you down. When you hear this voice, think the command "STOP!" Then give yourself positive messages, such as "I can handle this!" or "I am good enough."

In the quiet of your mind, you can receive wisdom about what is good for you, and then go on to create this reality. In fact, we need such quiet time to create and maintain a reality that will resonate with who we truly are. When we don't make time for it, our Inner Critic beats us up for having lives that don't seem to be working for us. And then stress caused by our perceptions impacts our lymphatic system, immunity and overall state of health!

Doesn't it sound right to you that in order to mute your Inner Critic, you need to purposefully stop and get off the roller-coaster of life for a bit each day? In the quiet of your mind, you can allow for the opportunity to see how your own good could unfold, as well as the good of others. It takes a peaceful mind to make wise choices. Plus, having a peaceful mindset in itself will rid you of the stress that creates self-blame and criticism.

So quiet your mind, and also observe all the good that you are! Come to understand that you (like everyone else) are doing your best in each and every moment. If you could do any better, you would! And it's only when you get rest, and create space for self-acceptance and a recognition of necessary changes, that the changes can appear.

♥ **A point to consider:** By silencing my mind, I will be able to make wiser decisions and rid myself of my Inner Critic.

♥ **Affirmation:** I can change my self-critical way of thinking.

♥ **A question to ask:** What other steps can I take along the road of self-support and self-acceptance?

*Responding is choosing
to take your power and use it
to reflect who you are inside.*

♥

6 Responding Vs. Reacting

Emotions are led by your choices and your responses. Are you responding or are you reacting? When you react, you allow a situation or another person to overpower you. It's a way of handing over your power and that choice is always toxic to our lymph system. For example: You're having a conversation with someone, and they are negatively judging your choices. Rather than responding with the word "I" and saying how you feel about being judged, you react by making the other person wrong, raising your voice in anger, and creating a circumstance where the other person has to defend themselves.

Responding is choosing to take your power and use it to reflect who you are inside. That's called emotional and mental "discipline" or "empowerment." With your actions, you're saying, "This is how I'm feeling about what's happening. You don't have to agree, however I need to express myself."

Reacting is about being at the mercy of someone else and saying that the other person is better, smarter, and more important than you are. However, since we're all exactly on the same level of life and there's no room for judgment, it's our duty to respond coming from who we really are – not from who the other person is.

If we were all meant to be the same, we would have been designed that way. Instead, each of us has absolutely individual responses to every single thing that ever occurs in our life. Respecting who you are is your reason for being alive. Don't go against that design! You deserve to let the world know the responses coming from your gut. When you do, you'll be honoring the flow that is YOUR FLOW OF LIFE, and this choice will also support your health.

♥ **A point to consider:** Empowerment comes from living and speaking my truth without judging myself or others.

♥ **Affirmation:** Responding rather than reacting allows me to live more effectively.

♥ **A question to ask:** If I honor myself, is there a need to react, rather than respond?

Oh, what a little break can do!

♥

7 Taking Breaks

To recharge your batteries, and maintain an emotional balance, you need to allow for a short or long break – escaping from your "stuff to do time." What a little break can do!... especially as far as your body is concerned. "Help! Give me a break," it is screaming. "Don't push me so hard that I become traumatized and off balance. Take me out of this business of pushing, never stopping, and instead stop to re-energize me. Take me to the place where I will be glowing."

For instance, you might head outside and notice the difference in how you feel. The actual "light" from above can transcend your low energy and lift you up! As this experience generates greater access to your clarity, you will attain the ability to be in union with your inner wisdom. Then the inner work triggers outer changes.

As part of your breaks, plan something entertaining that you'll look forward to doing. EXCITEMENT and UPLIFTMENT will help you to stay positive and maintain a good outlook. This also supports the flow of lymph, providing the movement necessary to bring on the HEALING.

During one of your next breaks, try this exercise... Begin by quietly writing about something that already positively affects – or would positively affect – you and your life. Then close your eyes and picture your mind and emotions as a room with the door slightly open. Nudge the door open and create "open mindedness." Begin to allow yourself to think about this positive thing expanding in your life, and hold onto that thought. Every time your mind starts drifting off into other places, gently bring yourself back to your chosen focus and see where your open mind takes you.

Opening your mind through the exercise will help balance you, your life, and your lymph!

♥ **A point to consider:** A break creates a clean and clearer perception of reality, and it supports the flow of life.

♥ **Affirmation:** Remembering to take breaks makes my lymphatic system and my entire being clearer.

♥ **A question to ask:** Since I now know that overdoing it keeps me stuck, doesn't it make sense to stop and smell the roses?

You can only depend
on yourself
to figure out
what feels best to you.

♥

8 Discovering What Feels Best To You

Each day, you deserve to do a practice that will give you a sense of inner balance. No one can choose what might be right for you. Why? Because each one of us will like something different.

You can only depend on yourself to figure out what feels best to you. For example, in the area of exercise, some of you like to walk, play tennis, do pilates, rebound, practice yoga, dance, go to the gym, golf, etc. For entertainment, some of you prefer movies, museums, a romantic dinner, a party, plays, art exhibits, concerts, a picnic, and on and on.

There are many choices that you have, and it is most important to look inside when you decide. When you are able to listen to that little voice inside, the answers will flow easily to guide you. However, there is no right and wrong. It all comes down to the question of what feels best to you, based on your own priorities.

I suggest that you don't ask everyone else what they think you should do, especially if you're going to take their advice and have it be the last word. That's only going to give you what they think you'd like to do. How can someone else know what's right for you? We can only know what's right for ourselves. If someone else offers their advice, it's best to listen carefully and see what's valuable, but then make your own choice. That way, you're the ultimate chooser of what is your best bet.

YOU *DO* KNOW WHAT'S RIGHT *FOR YOU!!!*

♥ **A point to consider:** If I look to others, I will never know what's best for me. Only what they think is best for me.

♥ **Affirmation:** I know what's best for me when I look inside of myself and respect the answer that comes to me.

♥ **A question to ask:** Can I trust myself to make my own choices and feel good about it, no matter what anyone else thinks or says?

Think of how nurturing it is
to just "tell it like it is,"
and set up a design
in your life that is actually
nurturing and feels right!

♥

9 Designing And Developing Boundaries

In her book, *Boundaries: Where You End and I Begin*, author Anne Katherine, M.A., provides an excellent definition of boundaries. She writes, "A boundary is a limit that defines you as separate from others..." You can know what boundaries are desirable for you by examining your feelings. By paying attention to how you feel and seeing what doesn't feel good, you can design and develop boundaries that take care of you and allow for your nurturance.

I'm quite sure that all of us can relate to a time when we definitely felt we didn't want to do something that a friend, lover, or family member wanted to do. And because we wanted the other person to like us, not be angry at us, and/or to be a good person, we went along for the ride. That was despite the fact that we *absolutely knew* that we didn't want to do this!

Alternatively, think of how good it feels to just "tell it like it is," and set up a design in our lives that actually is nurturing, and feels right... an approach that makes our body and mind say, "YES! YES! YES! Thank you for honoring me, since we are your best friends and will remain there for you when you are there for yourself."

When you know what you want to say to another person about a situation, I suggest that you speak the words first to yourself and then to the other involved in the picture. That way, guess what happens? You will be supporting not only your body and mind, but also your lymphatic system once again. Your lymph won't be stressed from your avoidance.

Yes, boundaries help your emotions and mind, and they strengthen your well-being. They also support a happy and healthy lymph system. So just say "YES" and mean it, and say "NO" and mean it!

♥ **A point to consider:** I am worth the effort of designing and developing boundaries to support who I am.

♥ **Affirmation:** Boundaries enable me to serve myself and others to the highest degree.

♥ **A question to ask:** Am I worth having boundaries so that I can be all that I am, rather than walking around frustrated and blaming others for it?

There is a bigger and better plan
for us
than we know.

♥

10   Trusting The Process Of Life

One perspective in life that encourages lymphatic flow is seeing every experience as an opportunity. I believe that since the beginning of time through today, there are reasons why every occurrence has come about. For example, perhaps you meet a new person who is very attractive to you, however they remind you of one of your parents. Thinking about the similarities, you realize that this person may have shown up to help you work through something incomplete in your relationship with that parent.

God (or the Universe, if you prefer) works in funny ways. There is a bigger and better plan for us than we know. Trust in the process of life can give you the ongoing faith that brings a more blissful existence and a healthier lymphatic system.

Have you noticed that the times that bring us the most challenge are those that make the biggest difference in our lives? Sometimes it looks like pain gives us much to gain. So know that when life is giving you events that push your buttons, something good is happening on another level. It's at these times that we must stop, look, and listen in order to see what the benefits are. Rest assured that you will see SOMETHING GOOD IS HAPPENING!

You're being tested, tried, and brought to new levels when experiences are pushing you this way and that. These new levels are your gift. You can fight this process, which will bring on more stress, or you can continue to go with it and receive the answers to questions that may have been getting in your way for some time.

YOU ARE ALWAYS IN THE LEARNING CURVE, SO WHY NOT GET INTO IT AND REALLY BE THERE? You will receive something and you deserve to receive the eventual goodness that the process of life has designed for you!

- ♥ **A point to consider:** I am gaining something with every experience that comes my way and I need to always keep that in mind.

- ♥ **Affirmation:** I will honor the processes that are given to me in life.

- ♥ **A question to ask:** Am I willing to stay in the process until I get the lesson or gift?

*The only thing that encourages self-worth
is when you take your life and own it.*

♥

11 Seeing Your Self-Worth

When you look to others for your self-worth, you're going to be disappointed. We all need to learn to see our own worth, as we are in the best position to understand our own gifts and strengths.

Without self-worth, our movement through life can become self-defeating. It's like God made us the way we are, and if we don't like it, we will send that negative message out into the world and that's what will come back to us.

Motivitional speaker Les Brown once said, "*Shoot for the moon. Even if you miss it, you will land among the stars.*" What Brown's message means to you, or me, or any person is that when you do what your heart leads you to do, you will land among the stars. In other words, when you believe in yourself, you follow your own lead. That in itself lifts you up and feeds your self-worth. And it allows your lymph to flow.

When you need a shot of self-worth, try listening to yourself and be the YOU that you are. This is acknowledging your uniqueness and not getting distracted by your fears of what others think of what you're doing, saying or thinking. Remember, even if we doubted our self-worth in the past, it's only NOW that matters. Each moment gives us an opportunity to see ourselves in a new light. An inner light shines when you appreciate yourself!

When you find yourself blaming others for what is coming back at you in the world, see that the outcome is based on what you contribute and your self-worth is a big part of the issue that is creating the outcome. Forget blame. The only thing that encourages self-worth is when you take your life and own it.

Of course, some of you may be faulting your parents or someone else who is close to you for your lack of self-worth, so let's look at that for a moment. If your parents were supported for who they really are and not who their parents would have liked them to be, they'd have the tools to use this parental attitude with you. However, if they weren't fortunate enough to have that kind of support, changing your sense of self-worth will be up to you. Now, in this work, it helps to choose FAITH. With faith, you can turn the tide and change the circumstance.

They say it's an inside job, and this is true, isn't it?! You can increase your self-worth – and each person's self-worth that you come into contact with – by being the good example. It's just that simple.

- ♥ **A point to consider:** I deserve an appreciation of who I am, since I'm unique and special like everyone else is.

- ♥ **Affirmation:** I can achieve a higher level of self-worth through trust and faith.

- ♥ **A question to ask:** Can I let go of my preconceived notion that it's someone else's responsibility to create my self-worth, or can I get over it and believe in myself on my own?

*Can you imagine a world
filled with gratitude?*

♥

Can you imagine a world filled with gratitude? A world populated with people who have the ability to see the glass as half full, rather than half empty? I can guarantee you that the lymph system flows better in someone with an attitude that is full of gratitude rather than a person who constantly complains.

So many times, I find myself asking, "What am I grateful for?" That's instead of "Why didn't I do this?" or "If only I hadn't done that!" It's very powerful to get into a grateful mindset. In fact, Oprah Winfrey did this in a way that she believes to have changed her life. She wrote down twenty to thirty things that she was grateful for every day. Oprah did this for three months, and it made a huge difference to her. Try it yourself. You'll be shocked at how much it will change your attitude.

BE GRATEFUL!!

I tried Oprah's gratitude exercise myself. And as I wrote the items down one day, I saw that I was focusing on all the good things that had happened. I didn't have time to focus on the negative things that would have normally drawn my attention. Suddenly there I was, noticing all the good during the day so I could add it to my list! My whole personality became lighter, brighter, happier, more confident, and more engaged in the moment. Plus my energy increased dramatically! My lymph was flowing well too as a reflection of my new focus. I was amazed!

I began to suggest that my clients make a gratitude list if they liked the idea. The ones that did it came back and said they were astounded. They felt better, had more energy, and experienced higher spirits! They definitely felt the difference.

Think of being grateful as the opposite of complaining, whining, blaming, feeling sorry for yourself, and just plain looking at all that doesn't come out the way you thought it should. Actually, if you have faith that your circumstances are the way they're suppose to be in order for you to grow and learn, you'll be grateful for the opportunity to experience life just as it is... and not how it is not!!

Here's something else to remember when you go through life passages that are painful and sad. It's alright to feel the feelings, acknowledge them, and let them be there. When it's all said and done, you'll experience plenty of gratefulness when you are on the other side of it!

- ♥ **A point to consider:** It's easy to see what does not feel good. However, I become a more powerful person when I'm grateful for what is!

- ♥ **Affirmation:** BE GRATEFUL. Be grateful. Be grateful.

- ♥ **A question to ask:** Would I experience more joy if I accepted life as a gift?

When your mind creates thoughts
of things, people and circumstances,
it draws those very things to you.

♥

13 Choosing Your Thoughts

Your choice of thoughts impacts your reality, including the state of your health. So switch a thought before transforming it into reality, unless it will be of benefit. DISCIPLINE your mind and emotions to work for you and your lymphatic health.

When your mind creates thoughts of things, people, and circumstances, it draws those very things to you. So this can work both for you and against you. If you expect to get sick because you're working too many hours and not getting enough rest, of course there you have it... you get sick! On the other hand, if you're dealing with a temporary heavy work schedule but are mindfully compensating with rest, exercise, a good diet and stress reduction, you're able to glide through the period while remaining healthy.

When you know that your thoughts attract what you'll have, you can become very powerful and quite supportive of your FLOW OF LIFE. You can become a conscious creator, rather than an arbitrary one. And one of the things you can help manifest is a healthy lymph system.

Gifts are given every day all the time. You can accept them or reject them. But you can only recognize the gifts that match your thinking. When you are able to acknowledge the gifts that present themselves, it moves you forward and supports the flow of the lymphatics.

So what's my message? Movement in life comes from your thoughts! They can either support your flow or impede it.

By the way, words work in a similar way to thoughts. You speak the words and then the words turn into your reality. So SPEAK WHAT YOU WANT, not what you don't want. It is your life. Say it the way you want it to be for YOU. You're your own boss and your own high priest.

♥ **A point to consider:** I run my own ship, so I need to watch where I guide my journey.

♥ **Affirmation:** I create my reality with my thinking.

♥ **A question to ask:** If I control my thoughts, what can I do differently to positively affect my reality and my lymphatic health?

What bothers you the most
about other people?

Could it be something
that bothers you about yourself?

♥

14 Being Bothered By Others

Why do others bug you? Let's take a look at this. When you are judging and not liking someone, could it be about something that bothers you in yourself? About a quality or behavior you dislike or feel deficient in? YES! ABSOLUTELY. It could be and *it is*!

When you're judging others, it means that the initial judgment and blame started with yourself. So notice when you don't like something about another person. Cradle that thought, and recognize the exact thing that puts you in a state of dislike for him or her. See that it is something which bothers you about yourself. Could it be that these people are offering you opportunities to work through your areas of personal challenge? DEFINITELY! They are your *gifts*!

"*Hmph! What a gift!!*" you might think. I sympathize! So here's an idea. How about using these encounters as good opportunities to use your sense of humor and laugh at life for giving you this person to help you grow? And as you go through the process of growth and work on lightening your load, the lymph will have an easier and easier time.

To get to the other side of a particular personal issue, embrace what makes you ill at ease about yourself and nurture yourself in this area that hurts. As in other parts of life, "what we resist" will persist. But once you embrace and work on whatever it is that's annoying you about yourself, you'll soon be able to see that you no longer have so much energy around it. And eventually the person who annoyed you will suddenly become *no big deal!*

Just think about it. You have the power to stop yourself from allowing others to bother you! Yes, when you start embracing yourself for all that you are, and stop being so self-critical, you will be able to stop being so hard on others. Then guess what? Your inner and outer flow will resume, and you get to let out a huge HOORAY!!

- ♥ **A point to consider:** Just think how lovely it is when you embrace who you are and how great it will be not to be bothered by others!

- ♥ **Affirmation:** There is much value in embracing what bothers me about others and therefore myself.

- ♥ **A question to ask:** When will I begin to let go of judging myself and start allowing others to be who they are without it bothering me?

Asking for help allows us
to see the beauty in life
and realize that there's good
to be had at all times.

♥

15 *Asking For Help*

It's surprising how many of us think it's weak to ask for help. Yet asking for help when you need it releases the pressure that builds up when you believe that you have to do everything by yourself. WHAT A RELIEF to feel O.K. about getting the help you need!! And the people who resonate with your request will feel honored to be of service.

Yes, it is a special gift to give the right person the opportunity to be of service. Just think about it. You would only ask someone who is special to you, who can do what needs to be done, and who allows you to show your vulnerability. It is somewhat like when someone wants to pay for your meal; it is a gift to the person giving, as well as a gift for you to receive. A plus in any event!

And there's an additional bonus to finding help. Your lymph system will be off the hook and no longer traumatized when you let go and ask for what you need, rather than worrying, fretting, and being stressed.

What is it that makes you think you can do it all? There is no one person who can do it all, and the sooner you find that out, the better off your life, your lymph, and your health will be. My dad used to say something to me when I thought that I couldn't take a vacation because none of my co-workers would do the work as well as I did. He'd comment: "Judy, no one is indispensable. Not even you!" This is a truth that changes your attitude and gives you freedom.

Know that whatever person you choose to help you, the exchange will be a gift to you and to them at the same time. It's about realizing that life goes on, allowing yourself to get unstuck, and giving yourself a chance to start moving ahead toward all the lovely things that you were meant to enjoy.

Asking for help allows us to see the beauty in life, to realize that there's good to be had at all times – but only when you're freed up and able to see it.

- ♥ **A point to consider:** No one is indispensable, and it is healthier and more fun to be a team.

- ♥ **Affirmation:** It's wrong to think that everything can be handled by one person.

- ♥ **A question to ask:** Can I see that letting go of my ego and asking for help when I need it or want it is a good thing?

Truth be known,
there is no need to push past
what is healthy
and appropriate for you.

♥

16 Respecting Your Emotional Speed Limit

We need to recognize the value of driving within our emotional speed limit, listening to our inner messages and honoring them. It's like driving a car. We can drive an automobile above the speed limit, but then we have to look over our shoulder to see if there's a cop nearby. We expect to get into trouble. We get stressed and so does our lymph system. In the similar way, when we don't pay attention to the speed limit recognized by our inner wisdom, we become stressed, look over our shoulder, and live at war with ourselves.

If a time comes when you feel pressed beyond the point of being balanced, this is a clue that you need to stop, look, and listen to your emotional needs. And what are your clues that you need time to scope out how to better respect yourself? Some common clues are anxiety, impatience, feelings of fatigue, etc.

At these times, assess what might be the best move to restore balance so that your mind and emotions can replenish. Is it a walk on the beach, a long relaxing bath, saying NO and meaning it, saying YES and meaning it, taking a few days off, visiting with a dear friend, reading a good book, or just plain doing nothing but staring out the window? What works for you?

Truth be known, there is no need to push past what is healthy and appropriate for you. So why would you do it? Pushing too hard may be your way of paying too much attention to the outside world. However, your first and foremost priority is your personal upkeep. Can't you just hear your body screaming. That's right!!!! It's screaming for your help. And your lymph system is suffering as well.

Respect your body, your limits, your needs, and pay attention!

♥ **A point to consider:** When my load gets too heavy, I need to back up, take a break, and respect myself.

♥ **Affirmation:** The best of all worlds is to be aware of what's too much and what's needed for balance in my life.

♥ **A question to ask:** What stops me from respecting, supporting, and listening to my body when the signals are so clearly being shown to me?

No matter what happened,
or is going to happen,
you're always offered the opportunity
to regenerate.

What a lovely thought!

♥

17 Regenerating Emotionally

The wonderful thing about life is that every moment is new. The past is gone, the future is not here yet, and what we have is the now. Know that no matter what happened, or is going to happen, you're always offered the opportunity to regenerate. What a lovely thought!

No matter what condition your emotional state and your lymphatic system is in, the opportunity to rejuvenate yourself is always available. Not to worry, we're designed to be renewed – both physically and mentally. So make yourself a priority!

Some examples of how you can emotionally support yourself are:

- ♥ Writing about your feelings and thereby releasing the emotional and physical tensions

- ♥ Exercising regularly (aim for five days a week)

- ♥ Staying flexible (physically, mentally, and emotionally)

- ♥ Using life as an "earth school" and seeing the value of each circumstance

- ♥ Being client

- ♥ Nurturing yourself

And how do we nurture ourselves? Everything that will stir your happy juices can be your right way. This is called a CHOICE. The endless possibilities include:

- ♥ Indulging in a lovely bath

- ♥ Keeping fresh beautiful flowers in view

- ♥ Relaxing with music you love

- ♥ Making special plans (a jazz concert, theatre performance, comedy show, crafts fair, day at the spa, etc.)

- ♥ Inviting a special person to share a meal, a talk, a walk, or a vacation

- ♥ Doing something that makes you happy each day

- ♥ Venturing out into nature

- ♥ Smiling at your face in the mirror and saying, "I love you!" (and meaning it!)

- ♥ Coming to your life and your days from the heart, because that's a place of softness, kindness, love, and gentleness.

Isn't it amazing that you have so many hours in the day, yet so often you'll hear yourself say, "I don't have time to do something for myself." Oh no, don't go there! You don't want the consequences. One day when you least expect it – if you don't take time for yourself – this life strategy could backfire, and your lymphatic system will be too tired to do its job of detoxifying the body. Just know that you are in control of your time, and therefore your health.

It's quite important for you to get that you have this power. After reading this information, you have the know-how of what it takes to rejuvenate your mind, spirit, and lymphatic health!!! So there! You can't argue with that – because it's true!

Take time for you!

- ♥ **A point to consider:** Now that I have ideas and tools for regenerating, I can do this.
- ♥ **Affirmation:** I will take time for myself, which will support my mind, spirit and lymphatic health.
- ♥ **A question to ask:** What are the things that nurture and rejuvenate me?

*Look for the beauty
and you will find it!*

♥

18   Seeing The Beauty Of Who You Are

Be your own best friend by looking at yourself and seeing the beauty in YOU. This might take special effort on your part. For if you're anything like me, you grew up always hearing about what you DIDN'T do or have – not what you DID do or have. Believe me, I see the disaster lurking in that type of negative reinforcement! However, there comes a time when it gets old to blame others for what they didn't know. What's important now is that YOU know that you're beautiful, no matter what! Look for the beauty and you will find it!!!

Turn the tide and quit being so hard on yourself. Look at all you have to offer. Pay attention to your beauty – inside and out! You were designed to be exactly who you are, so that has to be good! To look like yourself, to feel like you do, to see things through *your* eyes, and to be proud and loving toward yourself – that's the ticket to being able to see the beauty in others. But you can only see the beauty in others to the degree that you can see it in *you*.

You set up the precedent. And when you can accept who you are emotionally, you will be supported lymphatically as well. Beauty then comes from your inside out. In fact, it will be overflowing.

Yes, there is a flow in acceptance, whereas blockage is created when you resist who and what you are. Doesn't that make sense? So be the beautiful real you, not the less-attractive "fake you" others want you to be. It's really none of your business what other people think you should be. We're all perfect creations – creations made of love.

Your degree of beauty and the condition of your lymphatic system will be a reflection of how you live your life. Are you appreciating your beauty – or not?

♥ **A point to consider:** The fact that I exist means I am a gift!

♥ **Affirmation:** By seeing the beauty in me, I can see the beauty in others.

♥ **A question to ask:** What are some of the beautiful points about me?

With distractions,
it's sort of like
having everything you want
in front of you
but no time to access
it into your reality.

♥

19 Emptying Your Life Of Distractions

By emptying your life of distractions, you create an opportunity to enter into your inner world and seek guidance. Yet, instead of taking this time, many people fill up their days with TV, phone conversations that go on and on, reading, the radio, and unending plans. You then cannot hear your own inner voice, or meaningfully think about creating your life as you would like it to be.

In addition, there are so many instances when interruptions or distractions can pull us away from something that is so meaningful. Later we realize that we shouldn't have allowed distractions to get in the way. Perhaps working on establishing simple boundaries would be a good way to support your life, your health, and your goals.

When you're not distracted, you are available to do and be. With distractions, it's sort of like having everything you want in front of you and no time to access it into your reality. Ask yourself this question: Can you honestly say that not allowing distractions is an important step toward a personal world of satisfactions as well as a healthy lymphatic system? *Absolutely*!!!

So become your own distraction and guide. Only you know the path and how you must clear the way in order to reach the destination of peace, health, and happiness.

- ♥ **A point to consider:** I have the power and courage to honor my time, and I value myself enough to make the rules.

- ♥ **Affirmation:** Distractions let me know that boundaries are needed.

- ♥ **A question to ask:** What type of distractions will you work on eliminating first?

If you had the choice
to do anything playfully,
what would it be?

♥

When you run out of work and "being busy time," you will be forced to PLAY. Playing is the ultimate in nurturing the mind and your lymphatic health.

Stop and think about the times when you've felt the best. I'll bet it wasn't when you were overworking and being stressed with too much to do. For me, the best times come when I take a moment and say to myself, "If I had a choice to do anything I wanted, what would it be?"

Try asking yourself that question. Then you might find yourself thinking, "But do I really have the choice to do *whatever* I want? And if I do, what's in my way?" "ME AND ONLY ME," your inner voice will reply. At that point, reality will set in, and PLAY becomes the option and the choice.

To each of us, play means something different. So list the types of experiences that you consider play. Then, each day, take one of the items on your list and give it to yourself. PLAY and see the joy that is on the other side. Do you think you'll be glad that you honored your playtime? I dare you to say YES!

Play can range from taking a bubble bath, to going to a movie, to preparing a gourmet dinner for some special person or group, to making up a fairy tale for a child, to reading, to going to a stage production, to walking in the woods, etc. For you, PLAY is what you decide it is. There is no such thing as only one way to play. You make the decision, and you reap the rewards!

To embrace this topic, we can take a lesson from a child, and become child-like in our enjoyment of play. Your greatest gift is to keep the child inside of you alive so that you stay young for a very long time. Perhaps even till the very end... *the choice is yours.*

♥ **A point to consider:** I can choose to play each day.

♥ **Affirmation:** By deciding what I will look forward to each day, I will be creating excitement.

♥ **A question to ask:** What are the things in life that I consider play?

Whatever made us think
that we have the right to judge ourselves
or anyone else anyway?

♥

21 Forgiving Yourself And Others

Have you ever gotten into a pattern of blaming someone else, and carried that around with yourself for years? I did. For many years, I felt that my dad could have been there more for me emotionally, physically, and affectionately. Guess what? Because of my hurt feelings, I developed the habit of withholding my truth and repressing my feelings and communication. This eventually contributed to damage of my lymphatic system.

I felt that if my dad couldn't love and accept me, I must not be O.K. I built a case against my dad and therefore wasn't able to be the real me. Because of feeling insecure and unable to live in my full expression, at the ripe young age of twenty-eight years old I got cancer.

Through the gift of cancer, however, I got to realize that we're all doing our best – and *so was my dad*. If he had known how to do things better at the time, he would have. I'd also like to share that I always thought my dad didn't love me, which I later found out was not at all the truth.

Making a decision on something you don't have the real answer to is a dangerous thing. Please take a moment and think about the times when you have come to a conclusion about someone based on no real facts, only your assumptions. Then let those assumptions go, think about what you did know for sure about the situation, and forgive yourself.

You now have a new outlook on assuming and forgiving. And knowledge can open doors we've never walked through before, or even knew existed! However, once you know, you know!

I had to forgive myself for all the damage that I had created for myself, and then I could forgive my dad. I found that forgiving is a powerful thing. In fact, it is freedom. Forgiving takes the weights off of you and the person you couldn't forgive.

Whatever made us think that we have the right to judge ourselves or anyone else anyway? You are always forgiven!!! So forgive and lighten up!

Here's how I learned the truth. At age 35, I went to my dad and expressed my feelings. I asked him why he didn't love me. I was shocked and touched by what he said. He told me, "Judy, you weren't my problem; it was me. I didn't love myself and accept myself. You represented all that I really wanted to be – outgoing, happy, and social." I was speechless, knowing that I had suffered all those years thinking it was *me* who was the problem. It had been my dad's issues all along.

Let me tell you something, that blew me away. *All those years* I assumed that I was the problem, that I wasn't good enough, that something was wrong with me, that I wasn't lovable. None of this was true. Can you imagine the pain I had set up for myself and it was all based on assumptions - *my own assumptions*.

So when you think it's all about you, GUESS AGAIN!!! Life is not personal. It's all about the person that has the issue. It's not about you! That one understanding alone will help support your lymph system, as it will have less toxic waste to clean up from toxic thoughts.

It's best to discipline your mind and emotions to forgive, so that you keep the lymphatic system from having to work so hard. When the lymph is overtaxed, it can't do its job as well. And this lesson is one that I learned the hard way – by getting cancer.

If you can remember that everyone is doing the best that they can, you can forgive all people in your life, including yourself.

- ♥ **A point to consider:** I am forgiven!

- ♥ **Affirmation:** I know that everyone is doing their best and deserves not to be judged.

- ♥ **A question to ask:** How will I begin letting go of my judgment and blame so that I can be free to forgive myself and others?

In an environment of SELF-LOVE,
you thrive.

In contrast, without SELF-LOVE,
you suffer, feel lost,
and can't see the magic of life.

♥

22 *Loving Yourself Exactly As You Are*

You were born to be yourself, and that's the purpose of your life. Indeed, it is our biggest and most important job on earth!

Life designed you to be exactly who you are, with your look, your likes and dislikes, your choices, your creative abilities, your strengths, and your weaknesses. You must always remember that there is no other YOU! Yes, you were meant to be exactly the way you are and to be appreciated as such!

When you learn to accept and love yourself, you can treat others with love. In fact, to love, honor, and obey yourself offers you an experience that can enable you to give the highest form of LOVE possible to OTHERS. You see, you can only LOVE others to the degree that you LOVE yourself!

To accept and appreciate yourself is to LOVE the creation of You! And you can count on this LOVE to lift you up, and to bring you to a higher place. In an environment of SELF-LOVE, you thrive. In contrast, without SELF-LOVE, you suffer, feel lost, and can't see the magic of life. Without it, you live in judgment and pain, and life becomes hard and difficult.

Consider this... Where there is Faith and Trust in a Higher Power – God or whatever belief resonates with You – there is acceptance for the way things are, including the way YOU are. It is Faith that allows you to know that Nature is perfectly designed – the flowers, the ocean, the sky, the animals, people, and most of all YOU! Life's big plan is to be glorified and respected. And at those times when all else fails, your own inner faith will care for you and set you free!

Now stop and appreciate ten things about yourself. I'll bet you can easily do this. Write the items down and post them in a place that you go to daily. You are given so much! It is good to acknowledge the good and quietly be grateful. In fact, you can't afford to ignore the beauty that you are! It's the very thing that makes you special and unique.

The main thing is to confirm your love for yourself – who you are, what you represent, and what makes you feel good about yourself and your life. By getting into doing the things that create joy, you offer yourself the opportunity to smile from the inside out. And your lymph will respond to the smile and get in the flow.

So stop, look, listen, and step up to the plate... *Your plate*. That's the one designed especially for you! Bring on the LOVE, and that love will spread like wildfire to reflect out to all you see and touch. You do make the difference!

- ♥ **A point to consider:** Life designed me to be who and what I am, therefore I am perfect.

- ♥ **Affirmation:** What I am is good enough.

- ♥ **A question to ask:** What will I do to start demonstrating to myself that loving me is the key to loving others?

Without the sun,
there is darkness;
with it, there is light.

You are like the sun;
you can bring out
the joy!

♥

23 Recognizing The Joy In Life

I want to remind you that when life is appreciated for all that it is, your energy is light and joyful. When you resist what life offers, it darkens your energy. Which choice do you make most often?

Life is a gift, but it can end at any moment. So make a point of enjoying the journey along the way. This will bring you joy and make for a happier experience of living.

I like to think that a smile is like the sun – for both can change your life. Without the sun, there is darkness; with it, there is light. Likewise, your smile and sense of humor are the things in life that bring out the sunshine. You are like the sun; you can bring out the joy. Choose to laugh, smile, have fun, and be joyful!

Joy lightens the load for you, for others, and for the lymphatic system. Your lymph system deals with cleansing out the toxicity that comes with trauma and darkness. Open up to joy. At the same time, you will be giving yourself an inner flow. Your lymphatic system will recognize, respond to, and reflect your joyful reality.

You make a difference on the planet and on your lymphatic system, especially when you open up to joy and let it shine. Bring out the real you and share it with all who you come in contact with. That's the joy of living!

Life is just full of things that bring us joy. Doesn't it just blow you away when you recognize all that Nature offers – the flowers, the trees, the sky, the ocean, human beings, animals? There is too much to list here. Life is a miracle, full of so much for you to be grateful for. I support you to take it all in, breathe deep, and be with the joys that occur moment by moment. Through your appreciation and joy, you will affect the planet in a huge way and also benefit your lymphatic health.

♥ **A point to consider:** There is much in life to rejoice about!

♥ **Affirmation:** Joy is created by my own appreciation of life.

♥ **A question to ask:** Can I be in the moment so that I can experience the joy in life?

*Your inner messages
are very powerful, and
they were designed for you!*

♥

24 Respecting Your Inner Voice

Have you ever heard that little voice inside suggest that you do something, call someone, go someplace, say something... and you didn't listen? We all have done that, and the very thing we heard in our mind was what needed to be done. Then we find that because we didn't listen, something that would have worked out for the highest good didn't have a chance.

Your inner messages are very powerful, and they were designed *for you*. These messages deserve your undivided attention. They are there for a reason, and only your trust and faith will allow you to move on them and find out what gifts they have to give.

Yes, to the degree that you respect your inner voice, you will be gifted. These gifts will come in many forms and show you the next steps that are most appropriate for you. Did you realize how powerful you are?

Places of peace, fulfillment, and empowerment come from your ability to accept who you are, and your inner messages are the clues. Your biggest ticket is YOU! Who else but you can hear and follow your lead in this way? What is fascinating about the brain sharing your intuitive thoughts with you is that this leads you to *your right path*.

When your higher power gives you the messages and you listen, you are co-creating your life. This will take you from feeling powerless and alone in your existence to allowing the incredible to happen. And then with Faith, you can know that you'll never walk alone again.

Whenever you co-create with your inner voice, the lymph system flows along just as you are flowing along. So by befriending the idea of co-creating, you are sustaining a relationship within your own being.

But there is even more to this. As you honor yourself with each choice that serves you, you are also serving everyone on the planet. For it's peace that you'll receive by honoring that little voice inside of yourself, and this in itself helps build a healer in others and a world without pain. Peace begins inside each one of us.

I invite you to follow your intuition and allow it to lead you to a peaceful place!

- ♥ **A point to consider:** Peace begins inside of me, therefore it is my responsibility to follow my own lead.

- ♥ **Affirmation:** Respecting and honoring my inner voice allows me to respect and honor others.

- ♥ **A question to ask:** Will I allow myself to trust my inner voice and think twice at those times that I consider ignoring it?

You have been given
the gift of life,
and serving is your thanks.

♥

25 Being Of Service To Others

Creativity in your life's design is a spiritual act, not an ego trip. You were put on earth to make a contribution and to live a life of good deeds. So discipline your mind. Write your script so you can be of service to others – and thus to yourself. Your lymphatic system will reflect your wise behavior.

You have been given the gift of life, and serving is your thanks. Living on earth is an honor, one that you can take for granted or acknowledge with service when circumstances allow for it. You can say, "Thank you for the opportunity!" which blesses you with the gift of giving.

Have you ever been in need and someone just appeared without you asking? Think about what it felt like. Feel the feeling, close your eyes, and be there for a moment. Tell yourself in silence what it was like for you. Then remember... this is a feeling you can give to another.

And when you serve, the return will be huge. Yes, the reward will be big, and the greatest feeling of all is when the person being served looks into your eyes and you know that you were given an opportunity.

The power of being of service to others ignites both the giver and receiver. Serving changes and shifts what was into a better place! There's real beauty in supporting and nurturing, which ultimately creates movement. Then that movement transforms stagnation into flow – in you and around you. Giving is being in the flow, and flow is the ticket to a healthy lymphatic system.

You need to know how to light the fire of life and turn that fire up. One way is by gently being there and making the moves when the opportunity to serve shows up. You know what being of service is like. From nothing, you make something happen!

- ♥ **A point to consider:** Serving is an example of thanks and appreciation.

- ♥ **Affirmation:** Giving to others supports the flow of my life, and therefore it is a foundation for my lymphatic health.

- ♥ **A question to ask:** How can I start serving others?

Affirming the many gifts of life
and the experiences
that are given to you
makes them real.

♥

26 Walking Through The Open Doors Life Offers You

As you begin to trust and love your inner mind – allowing it to be your guide – you step in the direction of your dreams. And life opens doors unexpectedly. Your job then is to accept these opportunities, acknowledge them, and go for it! When you do this, the lymphatic system follows your flow and happily moves out the toxins to clear your body and support you with new energy so you can bring in the new.

Affirming the many gifts of life and the experiences that are given to you makes them real. Without acknowledgement, there is no reality. It is your view of what happens that makes it solid or not. So trust what life offers and follow that journey – it will add so much to your life!

Actually, it's your duty to yourself and to God (or the Universe, if you prefer) to go through the doors that open up for you. There's a reason the doors are there, and that reason will only be exposed if you open the doors and walk through them. Examine these potential experiences and see life as a "glass half-full." Get the most where the most can be gotten. Be grateful for the open doors. See the benefits!!

- ♥ **A point to consider:** Open doors are offering me an opportunity.
- ♥ **Affirmation:** There is always good where opportunities abound.
- ♥ **A question to ask:** How can I begin to follow and trust the doors that open up for me?

Recharge or not,
it will come back to you big time.

You can go either way,
for better or worse.

♥

27 Getting Rest, Sleep And Relaxation Time

REST, SLEEP, and RELAXATION support your emotions therefore they also increase the health of your lymphatic system. This trio gives you energy and clarity, and it allows you to be able to conduct your life in a self-supporting way.

For instance, when you are lacking sleep, you can't see things as clearly as you'd like. You could have a tendency to be picky, cranky, and short in patience and temperance. There is the vast possibility that you will judge, blame and argue.

So what the heck, you might as well give your body, mind and lymphatic system what they want. Why not? You will have nothing to lose and everything to gain.

You will then have the insight to see your own worth. You will be strong and rested and able to deal with your life without excessive emotional turmoil. You will shine and show your best self. In contrast, if you don't take care of yourself, you will be dispersing the worst of yourself out into the world.

Whatever you choose to give to yourself, it will come back to you big time. You can go either way, for the better or for the worst.

- ♥ **A point to consider:** My view of life is softer when I am relaxed.
- ♥ **Affirmation:** Rest is a necessary thing.
- ♥ **A question to ask:** What stops me from resting and relaxing?

*WHO you are being
is what matters...
not what or how much
you do.*

♥

28 Developing Your Character In The Script Of Life That You're Writing

It's a good thing to remember that you're a work-in-progress. Transformations in your character will unfold for the rest of your life.

As your script of life is created moment by moment, it's good to be aware that BEING the person you were designed to be is far more important than the doing. In other words, WHO you are being is what matters... not *what* or *how much you do*. So as you pay attention to your character each day, monitor yourself and see what you're being – don't just do while overlooking the way you're acting.

Write your best script. At the same time, be aware that when you're being an example of a person you like or don't like, it can become apparent to you through the condition of your health. If at any given time, you're not feeling well, recognize that a personal assessment is in order and a redesign of your life is needed. This is true because your lymphatic health is a mirror of you. After you make adjustments and your lymphatic system is working properly, you'll feel healthier.

And when observing your character, you'll become aware of both the beauty that you portray and the areas of challenge in your script of life. Shift the script you're writing to address these needed changes as well.

Now your script of life has a new view of how you make a difference in your inside and outside world. Keep making adjustments, and keep writing THE BEST SCRIPT FOR YOU!!

♥ **A point to consider:** I have the power to develop and re-design my movie each moment.

♥ **Affirmation:** My character creates the outcome of my health and life.

♥ **A question to ask:** What changes do I need to make as I begin to polish my character?

Think about what happens
when you check out
a situation
from a place of judgment,
rather than compassion.

It stops the flow.

♥

29 The Role Of Compassion For Ourselves And Others

Developing COMPASSION FOR YOURSELF creates the opening to experience it for others. It allows you to feel empathy for yourself and at the same time listen to these feelings.

The real heartfelt moments come when you are touched by an inner experience, or by someone else's experience. In fact, compassion is *the opening up of one's heart*, and it allows the lymphatic system to open, flow, and move at the very same time.

Your behavior either comes from a place of judgment, or from compassion. Think about what happens when you check out a situation from the perspective of judgment and decide which way you are going to respond. Your judgment stops the flow, produces stress, is not supportive, and creates blockages, both lymphatic and psychological. We were never given the right to be judgmental of ourselves or others. Therefore, choose to be compassionate. With this choice, you will be following the flow of life, and giving back to yourself and others.

Every situation is worth happening on some level, and it is up to us to find the gift in it. You can do it! It's your gift to have and to hold. So when you find yourself being judgmental, soften your stance, loosen up, and choose compassion.

To embrace messages that come from the unknown or from any source – be it a person, book, experience, movie, strangers, etc. – is also to be COMPASSIONATE. It's acknowledging that this source is there for you. Or if you give of your time and attention, it is having compassion and being compassionate. Compassion of all types supports lymphatic health, along with a feeling of well-being.

Being compassionate is a soft place. A place that feels like clouds in the sky or a baby's smooth skin. It is lovely and rewarding for the following reasons:

- ♥ Releases stress
- ♥ Supports flexibility
- ♥ Has a positive purpose
- ♥ So called "problems" are seen as opportunities
- ♥ Nurtures us
- ♥ Softens the rough edges
- ♥ Can release suppressed emotions
- ♥ Helps us to make wise decisions
- ♥ Acknowledges yourself and others
- ♥ Keeps an open mind
- ♥ Is an opportunity
- ♥ CREATES LYMPHATIC FLOW!

Look for how you could be more compassionate this very day, and enjoy the benefits!

- ♥ **A point to consider:** Choosing compassion adds something positive to all circumstances.
- ♥ **Affirmation:** Being compassionate is being in the moment, listening, having an open mind, and finding the gift in all circumstances.
- ♥ **A question to ask:** Can you remember that compassion is always available and all you have to do is choose it?

It is peaceful to relax into life,
to be open to what is.
Then havoc comes to us
when there is a
lesson to learn.

♥

30 Peace Vs. Havoc

Peace begins with a commitment to yourself and God (or a Higher Power). You create space for Life to fill and stop working so hard to have things be the way you think they should be. It is peaceful to relax into life – to be open to *what is*. Then havoc comes to us when there is a lesson to learn, and we will be blessed.

With this power, you are letting God and letting go. You are living out the creation and the enfoldment of what life has for you *personally*. At the point where there is no bad or wrong, you can choose to know that what comes in front of you is for your higher good.

What havoc brings is the opportunity to see a new way to experience life; this is something we could not get to on our own. Life has given us circumstances that may be uncomfortable to show us how to view things in order to change our way of being in the world.

This is a good thing!

Havoc or chaos – when there is no judgment – is neither good nor bad; it just is. This is what letting go of resistance is all about. You let go, transcend the moment, and allow life to be. At that point (and when we accept life in this way), the world becomes a peaceful place. Living without judgment and blame, you enable yourself to arrive at greener pastures. And you take your lymph with you wherever you go... so when you let go, you support this inner flow too.

When you can turn havoc into peace, it is healing *in every way*. You imagine peace and peace then prevails. How powerful you are! Your thoughts and your actions take you to the place where you were leading yourself.

When you realize you can do this, you see that you have a choice of havoc or peace at any moment. You choose, you create, and then you experience the positive outcome – *the gift*.

In my life, I was given the gift of Cancer. Yes, that time was full of havoc... however, I decided to scout out the avenues to learn the lessons that I needed to receive (which came because I hadn't been able to get there on my own). These lessons changed my life, my mind, and my lymph for the better!

- ♥ **A point to consider:** When I trust that what I am given is for my higher good, I will be supporting my flow of life as well as a healthy lymph system.

- ♥ **Affirmation:** Letting go of resistance creates a peaceful mind, body, and lymphatic system.

- ♥ **A question to ask:** In what areas of my life do I need to let go of resistance in order to gain peace and to support my lymphatic flow?

If you can't eliminate the stress,
change your reaction
to it!

♥

31 Choosing Our Response To Our Circumstances

Try this out for size. There are two people who are experiencing the same situation. Let's use the example of moving their living quarters. One is resisting the move, and feels uptight, scared, really shaky and cranky. The other is feeling an excitement about the new adventure and what it will bring – the new people, new environment, new feelings, and a new beginning!

Now why am I bringing this up! Well, because it's not important what happens to you. What's important *is how you respond.*

You always have the opportunity to see the glass as half empty or half full. Sit down for a bit and make a list of the circumstances in your life right now. In one column, list the circumstances that seem half empty and on the other side list the half full situations. Are you surprised at your responses?

Can you see that your thinking can make a difference in how you experience a circumstance? It creates your life, your attitude, and your lymphatic health. WOW! This is a big one! Affirm that you will see this truth in every condition of your life!

Perhaps it's a good time to examine your life and see clearly how your responses and attitude create the outcome. Say you have a business, and the business is flourishing and moving forward in a big way... and then it slows down a bit. Well, there are two ways to go here. You can panic and stress yourself, your cells, and your lymphatic flow, or you can trust that things have slowed down for a reason. Possibly you need the time in order to review, reorganize, catch up, and make the necessary adjustments that come with a growing business. It's called "time to take time." Yes, you can choose to freak out, or you could see that there is something to be gained by the circumstance. What a concept!

If you can't eliminate the stress, change your reaction to it! You are the sunshine of your mind. You determine how you view your state of life. Choose the glass half full! Heal your life, and keep your lymph healthy! You have all that it takes!!!

- ♥ **A point to consider:** It's not what happens to me that matters, it's how I respond to what happens that makes the difference.

- ♥ **Affirmation:** Every thought creates my life and my lymphatic health.

- ♥ **A question to ask:** How will I begin to reassess the circumstances in my life to see that there is a response that supports me and my well-being?

*Kindness has
the ability
to create happiness
wherever you go.*

♥

32 Showing Kindness

The glory of acting out of kindness is your gift to yourself. Why? Because when you act out of kindness, it is a reflection of how you feel about and act toward yourself. In other words, to be kind to others, it is first necessary to have the experience of liking yourself, being good to yourself, and loving yourself. So when you look at how you treat others, it is a direct indication of how you are with yourself.

Do you like how you are? Are you proud of yourself and respectful of who you are? As you answer these questions, you are given the opportunity to see what you might like to begin doing differently. It's all so easy when you realize how powerful you are. All you need to do is to be kind to yourself. The rest is a piece of cake.

Now look into your past. What gave you peaceful energy, an abundance of joy, and made your heart sing? Yes, those experiences that created a glow from the inside out are the ticket! That glow comes when you find life stimulating. So see life as an upper. Glowing is really a good thing!

And what happens to you when your feelings are elated? Yes, you guessed it. You want to jump, dance, sing, and move. That feeling is the stimulation that makes for good health, as well as good lymphatic movement.

And what about being kind to others? When you have the opportunity to offer even the smallest favor without being asked and you're the instigator... OH BOY, that's a treat to the largest degree!

When kindness becomes your friend, it has the ability to create happiness wherever you go. You shine from the inside out, and your lymphatic system is relaxed enough to move out the bad and bring in the good. Hail, Hail to KINDNESS!!

♥ **A point to consider:** In order to show kindness, it is imperative to be kind to myself.

♥ **Affirmation:** My ability to show kindness depends on how I treat myself.

♥ **A question to ask:** Do I think enough of myself to be kind out in the world?

It's all about working together
to have experiences
that feed everyone –
not depriving any person
that's involved.

♥

33 Working As A Team Player In Relationships

In relationships, it's a team approach that brings balance to your existence. This is accomplished when you work with yourself, are yourself, tell your truth, choose your likes and dislikes, and love, honor, and obey your true self at all times. From this place and only this place can you honor others.

Let's take the checker at the supermarket. Even in that brief period of time that you share, you have a short relationship. Are you imclient with the person or do you feel grateful and pleased that you are being taken care of? Is the checker pleasant to you or is their energy one of "I hate being here"? Both you and the checker are probably treating each other as you are treating yourselves. Life is not personal! People act out their own stuff.

However, what you want to do is to act with more consciousness. For example, let's say there is a decision to be made and it involves someone else and yourself. The magic that creates an outcome that will feed both people comes from co-creation. In straight terms, you both sit down, say what you want, listen to each other, and work out the goal that will match up with both of your wishes. The feeling is "I care about you and you care about me, and we co-create together." As you create in this way, the brain-waves signal the body that all is O.K. "on the Western Front." The body then can relax, the lymph flows, and you gain a glow that comes from within.

So what's the answer? It's all about working together to have experiences that feed everyone – not depriving any person that's involved. When you can do this, you honor others for who they are and join forces to create a team. Meanwhile, being open and non-judgmental will protect you from your own negative energies, and being in this state will support you to engage with others in a way that offers a view of the real you. When you open up, there is a world of relationship that will and can be fulfilling – whether the relationship is for five minutes, five hours, five months, five years or five decades!

All it takes is to open your heart with loving gestures and kindness. Then you'll find that there is power in relationships. There is power in more than one. Relationships create the circumstances and the outcome to everything we do. So everyone we deal with – in every moment of every day – is important.

You have the power to engage in healthy relationships at any given moment that you decide to honor, listen to, and treasure yourself. Go ahead... make it happen! You can do it!

- ♥ **A point to consider:** It takes self-love to create loving relationships and teamwork.

- ♥ **Affirmation:** I honor myself and others in my relationships.

- ♥ **A question to ask:** Where in my life would I like to let go of judgment and blame so that I can experience teamwork and lymphatic health?

*To listen
is to love
and to cherish.*

♥

34 Listening As A Tool

You gain something huge when you listen. You lose something huge when you don't. Listening to yourself and following the messages of your inner self will always guide you to delicious places of truth, personal growth, and important movement. But it's when you learn to experience other hearts and souls as well that relationships flower, grow, and are fulfilling in the most beautiful ways.

In fact, relationships work to the degree that you listen. In order to be a team and have balance, the art of listening is a needed part of the relationship. People love to be heard and love to be listened to. It is the way we connect on a deep level. Listening creates intimacy with others, and it allows relationships to flow smoothly.

Consider carefully how you listen. If you are wanting to be heard rather than to hear, you are not being there in the moment. You are somewhere else, and there is no continuity or relating. At that point, you are wasting your time, and the time of others that are in your company. In addition, you have created a trauma to your lymph system, which is responsible for your inner flow.

Yes, listening is a power tool. It's through listening that we share, express, love, expose, show passion, open our hearts, and take ourselves to tender places that are real – oh so real! To listen is to love and to cherish.

- ♥ **A point to consider:** It takes listening to get what is to be gotten every step of the way.

- ♥ **Affirmation:** Listening provides the opportunity to have clarity.

- ♥ **A question to ask:** What will remind me to listen to myself and others in order to be open to what I need to hear?

Share yourself,
bare yourself,
and also share your fun,
your love, your learning,
and your empathy.

♥

35 Being Willing To Share

The art of sharing is the part of relationship that feeds your Soul. Ask yourself and then tell yourself how it feels to share your love, support, adventures, truth, intimacy, and time. But don't confuse sharing with being comfortable. It's not always so.

Sharing a relationship involves your body, mind and soul. When you are good to yourself and share your innermost gifts, you bring closeness to the relationships you develop.

When you share, you care! And when you care and share, you send tender messages of kindness to yourself – and to others. This ultimately will positively impact your lymphatic system.

For example, maybe you were able to open up and let go of what you were holding back. You allowed yourself to shine, become known, and let the other person into your world. This was a time of opening up some of those hidden places inside of yourself, and you were then able to let go of the tense feelings that were connected to them. The act of sharing allowed nervous energy to move, and this movement got reflected in your every cell and lymphatic vessel.

Sharing your inner self is one of the most rewarding aspects of sharing. It assists in unblocking the areas of your life that were full of fear. It allows others to be closer to you to support who you are, and to love the person that you are. Consider this... your uniqueness is what makes you who you are. Doesn't it make sense that to be loved you first need to share yourself?

So share yourself, bare yourself, and also share your fun, your love, your learning, and your empathy. You will be caring for yourself and your lymphatic system at the same time.

♥ **A point to consider:** Sharing is caring.

♥ **Affirmation:** I share the real uniqueness of who I am with others.

♥ **A question to ask:** Can I let go of my self-judgments so that I can share all of who I was designed to be?

Truly happy people
with balanced lives
spend a minimum of
two hours a day on themselves.

Does this
surprise you?

♥

36 Spending Time With You

Do you take time to have a relationship with yourself? Are things like talking on the phone or watching TV getting in the way of your "for yourself" time? Taking time means filling a space with relaxation and a smooth energy that results in self-enjoyment and rejuvenation. This time that you give to yourself also supports a healthy lymphatic system.

So when you are planning your day, fit yourself in there. Take time to do the things that allow you to feel good, look good, and connect to your inside self. Such time makes it easier for you to see how you tick... to understand what works or doesn't work for you... to obtain clarity about those areas of your life that are foggy to you. Can you imagine giving yourself the time you need to feel loved and cared for? The time you spend with yourself will show up when you are out in the world.

Truly happy people with balanced lives spend a minimum of two hours a day on themselves. Does this surprise you?

I'm sure that every one of you knows of ways to nurture yourself, feed yourself, strengthen yourself, and make yourself feel like the best you! Also, taking time will allow you to become aware of what you are proud of and have faith in about yourself, and it opens the door for the outside world to see too. You can only share yourself with others to the degree that you get to know who you are. But when your inside world is known, nurtured, and loved, you will shine like a bright star in the sky.

Finally, spending time with yourself will help you to let go of trying to be someone other than who you are. Take the time to know yourself! You will not be sorry. You will, instead, truly open up to a new you... a you that you can appreciate.

It takes time to develop a relationship with yourself, just like it takes time to build any intimate relationship. Give yourself the gift of time.

♥ **A point to consider:** You are worth the time! You are God's gift!

♥ **Affirmation:** The time I give to myself can help energize, support, and heal me.

♥ **A question to ask:** Can I accept how powerful providing time for myself can be?

*Love yourself enough
to begin adding or subtracting
whatever it will take for you
to bring balance to
the life you have now.*

♥

37 The Need For Balance

As Dr. Patricia Fitzgerald wrote in the Foreword, a common comment in our society today is "I'm so busy!" What is this saying? One thing that I believe is that it's a call for BALANCE. So here's a reminder. Take time for yourself and for your relationships. When you do, your relationship with your every cell, your mind, your emotions, your lymphatic system, and your total well-being will respond positively.

A good exercise would be to write down a common day in your life. Examine it, and ask yourself, "What do I need to change in order to have a balanced life?" Then answer yourself by writing your answer down. Love yourself enough to begin adding or subtracting whatever it will take for you to bring balance to the life you have now.

Don't be hard on yourself for what your recorded day or the past might look like. Today is the first day of the rest of your life. Make it a new beginning! Give yourself the gift of *now*. Then hug yourself and realize that *you* are a GIFT!

Let's look at the need for balance in the way people eat. Someone who is busy might pick up some fast food for lunch or dinner. Of course, there are no organic raw vegetables or fruit in this meal. Oh yes, the fast food fills them up, but what about their health? It can suffer the consequences as was evidenced in the movie, *Super Size Me*. What about taking into consideration that each person deserves a balanced meal, with live organic food incorporated? Plus time to sit down in a relaxed manner, thinking enough of yourself to enjoy the taste and yummy feelings that come with nurturing the body with nutritious food?

The never-ending job that your magical lymphatic system and body perform depends on you. You are the catalyst for the quality of your day, status of your health, and level of your satisfaction with life.

So design your time for balance. If you take time to appreciate life, smell the roses, get to know yourself and others, a certain clarity will occur. Good for YOU!

Taking time allows the brain, heart, and the body to connect and experience the moment. In the moment is where everything happens. If you are too busy and are always thinking about what you need to do or what you didn't do, you miss the now and will never get that moment again.

- ♥ **A point to consider:** It is honoring to myself, my health, and my relationships to design a balanced daily regimen.

- ♥ **Affirmation:** There is plenty of time to live a balanced life, and I take the time!

- ♥ **A question to ask:** What will support me in designing a balanced life?

Time, Time, Time.

There's no lack of it.

*So why not have
a new view of time?*

♥

38   *You Have All The Time You Need*

Time... All you have is time. Time, Time, Time. There's no lack of it, and yet people walk around feeling like it's scarce. They say I'm too busy to see my family, take care of myself, be quiet enough to know who I really am, exercise, go out with my friends, be creative, have a relationship, see my kids, eat healthy, and on and on!

Just remember, time never ends. It's always available! So take advantage of the freedom that time gives you. It's free; there is no lack of it. Doesn't that just give you a new view of time?!

You are in control of the time in your life. You can even waste time and feel good about it. Time is yours to do with as you please. Just make sure you *are* pleased. The world is filled with all the time you need.

So take the time to open the heart that is hurt, to make things right, to do all the things you need to do to take care of yourself. Be your own best friend. Tell yourself what choices feed your life and your heart. Choose to live each moment like it is your last. Take the time to tell yourself that you're OK being the person you were designed to be. Tell those that you love how you feel, smell the roses, watch the sunset, touch a baby's soft skin, spend time with elders, share your unique thoughts, trust and have faith. You have the time to do all these things and more!

Do yourself a favor, and please get the fact that time has no limits. If you believe you have no time, the issue is that you *take no time*. Just remember that if you take time for your priorities, you are feeding your inner priorities as well. Your lymphatic health reflects the amount of time that you allot to taking care of your body, mind, and soul.

What happens when you don't take time for the things in life that feed you, nourish you, and honor you? Life feels frustrating, depleting, tiring, stress-producing, unhealthy, draining, lonely, depressing, and you suffer the consequences that only time can heal. Doesn't it make sense to pay attention?...to give up doing the things that end up being the cause of neglecting the real priorities... to focus on the things that make a difference? Only you have the power to light up your life!

Taking time will not only feed you, but your other relationships as well. It is the food that creates a trusting, solid, nurturing love... which takes time.

Time also allows you to receive the joy of what taking time gives you.

Give yourself the gift of time.

- ♥ **A point to consider:** Time is my own. I can do what my intuition guides me to do with it.

- ♥ **Affirmation:** There is no lack of time.

- ♥ **A question to ask:** What gets in my way of doing what my heart and my soul tell me I am here to do?

When you have something to say,
tell it like it is!

You'll feel free and light,
and help any situation
in any relationship
by being you.

♥

39   *Telling It Like It Is*

Tell it like it is. Say what's so for you! It will help to say words without judgment and blame. Words create your reality. So say it the way you'd like it to be, but with a "soft around the edges" approach and not to purposely hurt anyone. Then, when you've said your truth, you will be in the moment and able to flow to the next place.

When you stuff it and don't speak your truth, your energy gets blocked, you are not able to be in the moment, and you miss the experiences that you are meant to have. In addition, your lymphatic system will reflect the stress caused when you habitually repress communication. Ultimately the body gets traumatized when you don't honor yourself enough to expose your truth.

Remember... in those times when you have something to say, tell it like it is! You'll feel free and light. Best of all, you'll help any situation in any relationship by being you... the you that you were intended to be. And whenever you are yourself, you gain strength, self-respect, and well-being.

Each one of us is designed to be unique. In sharing your one-of-a-kind self with others, you deliver and receive the lovely gift of relationships that are built on trust and love. Just keep in mind that how you are with yourself – and whether you do or do not communicate about your true feelings – designs the way you are with others. In fact, the degree that you let yourself be known is the degree that you are able to give and receive love.

When you tell your truth and someone loves you for all that you are – that is what unconditional love is about. Everyone wants it, and it is yours to have if you agree to let yourself be and shine like the star that you are.

How do you say your truth without putting the other person or people on the defensive? First of all, when you use the word "I," rather than "you," you can say anything you want without judging, blaming, or making the other person wrong. When you start a sentence with the word "I," what you are doing is letting the other person know how you feel. How can someone make you wrong for how you feel? However, the moment you point a finger at the other person and blame them, the natural reaction is to become defensive. It is the way of all people.

Interestingly, true love can only be gotten through the truth. If you are withholding the truth, love is not an option. Only when you have faith and trust in yourself enough to be honest and open, can someone else have faith and trust in your love and loving you. Doesn't it make sense that it's only if you let yourself be known, that others can appreciate your unique self? It is the way... the only way to have a solid foundation with anyone.

To simplify "telling it like it is"... listen to how you feel, look at how you feel, experience how you feel, then say it!! The truth will transform you. Growth is the process of replacing lies and repressed communication with truth. By honoring your messages from within, you allow yourself to be okay, you share the real you, and that very thing opens the space for others to know you and love you.

Be you! Let yourself be known. Tell it like it is!

- ♥ **A point to consider:** Telling it like it is – it's the way for each of us.
- ♥ **Affirmation:** By saying my truth, I am honoring myself, others, and my lymphatic health.
- ♥ **A question to ask:** What fears do I have that stop me from saying my truth?

As you begin to
swing along and be the you
that you were created to be –

and have that be
alright with you –

you will be in the flow.

♥

40 Being In The Flow

How do things flow to you? Don't they need a portal or a door to enter, and one that is open and receptive? It's the same with any area of life, be it a relationship, food, or an action. Therefore, listen to the advice of ancient Chinese philosopher Lao Tzu, who tells us: "*Be really whole... and all things will come to you.*"

What makes you whole? What supports your body, mind and spirit? What keeps your lymphatic system flowing? It is your ability to be in touch with your own feelings, to follow your own lead, and to experience whatever is in front of you. That's what creates the pure you.

Have you ever felt down and out of sorts, and you just wanted to just go to a place that felt nurturing? And once you made a choice for yourself that filled that bill, you were soon once again "in the flow." When you listen to that little voice inside you and follow its instructions, you get in the flow. Its guidance will assist the inside and outside of your body to move to the next place.

Be your own companion and friend; trust yourself and listen to yourself. As you begin to swing along and be the you that you were created to be – and have that be alright with you – you will be in the flow. And when you are in your own flow, it feels right.

Only you know what creates your flow, and getting in touch with this knowledge gives you the power to support yourself. You can feel it when you're in the flow, because when you are not there is resistance, anger, blocked energy, repression and weakness. It is a positive thing to go with the flow, even when it takes you through the dark side to get to the bright side. Honor your process. Perhaps, right now, you need to work through the blocks to create an easier flow.

It is no secret that when you feel good, the whole world can feel it and see it. So go inside, and embrace the place you are coming from, rather than resisting it. GO WITH WHAT IS AND THE FLOW WILL FOLLOW, TAKING YOU TO WHERE YOU WANT AND NEED TO BE!

♥ **A point to consider:** Blocked energy can be released by embracing it.

♥ **Affirmation**: I am worth the effort it takes to discover my natural flow.

♥ **A question to ask**: Doesn't it feel good when I acknowledge my personal choices, and respect my flow of life?

Love IS the answer.

♥

TO LOVE OR NOT TO LOVE... there is no question. In the short and long of it, LOVE indeed does conquer all. There is one purpose that we were put on this planet for and that is to LOVE ourselves, each other, and all that lives and breathes on this earth. The body, mind and soul respond positively to love. Love *is* the answer. It is the one thing in life that offers a healing effect whenever it is experienced. For example, love supports the lymph system in giving us the gift of a healthy life.

LOVE feeds the soul. It gathers all the good and spreads it around like butter on a baked potato. LOVE makes a dark moment feel better. LOVE caresses your body, mind and soul with a gentle touch of energy that changes everything for the better. LOVE has no limit, no request for return. LOVE only has love. And LOVE – being your most powerful gift – cannot require an equal return. LOVE is by itself a return.

The challenge you have is that sometimes you construe LOVE as being romance, or being in lust, or being something else. In truth, LOVE is always all and everything good.

LOVE yourself first, and love for others and other things will come from that place. Soon you'll discover that LOVE comes in all shapes, sizes, colors, and dimensions. You'll notice that different cultures express LOVE differently – in food, clothing, music, dance and history. Yet they are all the same LOVE.

In life, you can express yourself in situations in all kinds of ways, depending on that particular event or circumstance. You always are in a choice mode as to how you decide to be. How might you respond? Some examples are aggressive, angry, loving, soft, positive, judgmental, forgiving, negative, defensive, etc. Choose to be *loving*.

Find the love when you are blocked or stuck, and it will heal your body, mind, emotions and soul. You are the gift. Love yourself and others. Approach life with love.

- ♥ **A point to consider:** When I follow the journey of life with Love, I know all roads will take me to where I need to go.

- ♥ **Affirmation:** Coming from a place of love positively affects my body, mind, soul and lymphatic flow.

- ♥ **A question to ask:** Can I embrace life's circumstances with Love, especially when I feel uncomfortable?

When someone doesn't
get who you are,
can you see that
it only matters
if you don't think enough
of yourself?

♥

42 Dealing With Challenging Relationships

When relationships get crazy and go on fire in your life, do you just blame the other person and act like you had nothing to do with the circumstances? Do you bury your head in the sand? Yet isn't it true that everyone that's involved has a part in what's happening?

Well, don't be hard on yourself. Instead, lighten up about the people who have been driving you nuts or who you've felt painfully powerless with. The Rolling Stones had it going on when they sang, "You May Not Get What You Want, But You Get What You Need." Don't you just love it!

Every person in your life is there for a reason. When things get hot and stuff hits the fan, don't we receive a healing after all is said and done? Haven't you noticed that the relationships that "plug you in" the most and drive you nuts are the ones that teach you more than any others?

For sure, these testy relationships ain't easy! But don't you find that when you embrace this person, rather than resist them, you get to change, grow and even get to find that you feel better eventually. And they suddenly grow and change in the same way! Earlier, when they were defensive, it was out of a desire to feel safe. Everyone just wants to be appreciated for what and who they are.

Just think about it! Haven't you had relationships where you tried to communicate with someone who doesn't think like you, doesn't have the same outlook on life, isn't interested in what you're doing on many levels... and yet you still keep cramming the same information their way over and over. Turn the tables and think what it's like when someone tries to make you agree with them or see things their way when you just don't. How annoying!

To change any relationship or scenario, you need to change your way of being with this person. In fact, make peace a priority in your life through learning new ways of being in relationship with *all people* at all times. Clearly, some people are in your life to teach you to be able to appreciate them, even though they have no interest in what you are doing, how you think, or what you look like.

These people make you realize that you are the only one who needs to love and accept who you are. Isn't it wonderful to get that it's none of your business what other people think of you? Especially when you get that you are the only one who can make you feel OK about yourself. When someone doesn't get who you are, can you see that it only matters if you don't think enough of yourself? Yes, that's a biggie – isn't it?

Family relationships or work relationships can veer toward this category of challenging. Can you keep the relationship from becoming challenged? One option is... *work with it, not against it.*

People show up to expand your world, and to heal your heart. When we can come from an appreciation of who they are and what they represent, don't they mirror back the same appreciation in return? Doesn't this feel a whole lot better than forcing people to be like you? Why not allow different views and beliefs just to be OK? Isn't it easier to just love people for who and what they are? People who are defensive and angry are really calling out for love, because they don't feel good about themselves, or perhaps don't feel appreciated. Maybe it doesn't look like that... but usually it's true.

Don't take life personally. Listen to what people have to say... they are always telling you about themselves. It's An Inside Job.

♥ **A point to consider:** I am responsible for my relationships and how they feel.

♥ **Affirmation:** My relationship with myself is what can change a challenging relationship into a healthy relationship.

♥ **A question to ask:** Can I accept myself and have that be the basis of harmony in my relationships, rather than depending on the acceptance of others?

When you're in a learning mode
and life slips you an unexpected curve,
being soft with yourself and others
makes the journey flow.

♥

43   Being Soft Around The Edges

By keeping to your truth and at the same time softening around the edges in your way of being, you will support the nurturing of yourself and others. When you notice that you are responding in a cutting or edgy way, think about a baby's skin or a soft warm fuzzy blanket and bring that feeling to the surface. BE SOFT AROUND THE EDGES. It is easy to say and sometimes challenging to portray.

Every time you get hooked into a way of being that is not coming from a soft place, just know that you can imagine a picture of softness and shift into that place. We are all on this planet to live in a world of PEACE. Since peace begins inside of us, we can make a difference in the ways of the world... each one of us. By softening your words and ways, there will be a positive reaction on the inside and outside of your being. It will affect your own LYMPHATIC SYSTEM AND WELL-BEING. As you affect you, YOU ARE AN EXAMPLE – therefore affecting all beings. YOU MAKE A DIFFERENCE!

The test will be when you are in a situation that is not in your comfort zone and you have a hard time turning your way of being to a soft and loving place. It is easy to be soft when things are feeling wonderful and life is rolling along. However, when you are in a learning mode and life slips you an unexpected curve, that is when being soft with yourself and others makes the journey flow. This is when you have the opportunity to assist the movement in your life and your lymphatic health.

You can all remember times when you've expected one thing and got another. Your reaction or response can easily be one of acting sharp, short and somewhat angry. This is called *resistance*... And resistance creates persistence. Therefore, allowing the softness to take over supports the change you want to see. Softly.... go with the flow and the flow will take you to a new and better place.

♥ **A point to consider:** Being soft and loving feels better than coming from a harsh, fearful and defensive place.

♥ **Affirmation:** From a place of empathy and love towards myself and others, I am supporting the constant flow of life and lymph.

♥ **A question to ask:** Are you grateful to be living in this world, so that acting and communicating from a soft and loving space is your reality?

To be open to taking things into consideration
is to be willing to grow and expand.

♥

44 Consider This, Consider That

Consider all the things that come to you, are around you, and all the people that you are in relationships with. Consider your thoughts, your feelings, your comfort zones, your uncomfortable places, as well as other people's feelings, thoughts, likes and dislikes. It is wise to be considerate, since what you do or don't do affects the whole planet, along with your own life and health. What you do or don't do comes back to you. So it's best to move through life with consideration. What goes around comes around.

STOP, LOOK, LISTEN AND LEAVE the space to consider all points of view. It could be that what is in earshot are the exact words or actions that can open you up to a new possibility. There are no accidents. You are meant to hear all words and see all actions... all the time.

Trust that if something or someone else is in your space, it is worth considering. It is what makes ideas expand, change, and evolve. What might have been just good, with new input becomes great! These are opportunities to allow others into your world to play.

If you think you know, you better know now that you don't know! To be open to taking things into consideration is to be willing to grow and expand. In contrast, not to be open, not to consider, is to be stuck. When you lack consideration, you are stuck in the thickness, rather than moving with the flow. You are playing small and missing out on the extraordinary joys of life. Consider that! Why not release the tension, and consider a life beyond your dreams? Note all the support and information surrounding you, and drink it up!

When you see life as an open road, you open yourself up for new opportunities, people, growth, and a world beyond your expectations. You will be on the healing path... an easier path... a path full of surprises. Consider that!

Consider trusting and having faith in what's happening. When you do, there is no reason to always be asking, "WHY did this happen?" The WHY doesn't make any difference... the truth is, it just happened. And the other truth is that everything that happens has its own beneficial reason. So consider looking at any circumstance and finding what makes it beneficial. This is a good thing, since there is a lesson in everything. Through consideration, you will find the lesson. Without it, you may miss your education. Best to find it, rather than lose it. Ignoring it now, you'll only have to learn the lesson at a later date.

Why not soften up, and honor and consider the path that you are on. All of these things lead to movement and flow. This is a GOOD place to be... personally and physically.

- ♥ **A point to consider:** Consider that if everything has a reason, anything that happens is a positive event.

- ♥ **Affirmation:** Having trust and faith opens me up to getting the gift of considering that every situation has something good to offer – whether it looks that way or not.

- ♥ **A question to ask:** What gets in my way when it comes to considering being open to life's journey?

Your entire being is happy
when you look for
and see what
there is to celebrate!

♥

45 Celebrate Yourself, Celebrate Life!

To celebrate yourself, you must stay in the moment, rather than being in the past or the future. The now is where you learn to listen to yourself. Then, in the moment, you may realize that there's a need to forgive yourself. Forgiveness is key in loving yourself, and with self-love, you are able to treat others to your love and joy.

I invite you to celebrate yourself... to celebrate the people in your life and all that Life gives you to experience. If you believe and trust and have faith, you get to celebrate. If you don't believe and are mistrustful and doubtful, you will be left out in the cold wondering what went wrong.

Celebrating enables you to be encouraged by all that is. It enhances your energy for moving from this moment to the next, and with movement and adaptability you unleash the lymph to move as well.

Celebration is the hoorah! and it goes back to traditions of our ancestors. Throughout time, people sang, danced, hugged, laughed, prayed, and carried on in celebration. As they did, joy took over. And just as joy enhances your outlook and uplifts you, so it is that the lymphatic system becomes a mirror of that same effect.

Imagine the many types of adventures that are there to celebrate in your world. The ultimate goal in your lifetime is to get in touch with your own celebrations and to go for it! For one person, celebrating will be hiking, painting, and having a cup of tea and a piece of fresh apple pie. For another, it's dancing, singing, or taking a grandchild for a walk.

It is your uniqueness that is truly the gift that has been given to each of you to invest in. To be willing to be unique is to be open to true inner satisfaction. And through the feelings of celebration, you soar to places that you never quite imagined you could experience.

I commend you for being YOU! I support you in CELEBRATING the YOU THAT YOU TRULY ARE! YOU ARE WORTH CELEBRATING – NO MATTER WHAT! And as you celebrate yourself, you give others the encouragement to celebrate themselves.

Your entire being is happy when you look for and see what there is to celebrate. Just as looking at a painting can bring you to new places in your mind, sitting under a tree can open you up to appreciating all that has ever been created in Nature. Isn't all of life worth celebrating – including you?

CELEBRATE!!

- ♥ **A point to consider:** The difference between being in a dark space or celebrating is what makes my life what it is.

- ♥ **Affirmation:** Celebrating positively affects my mind, spirit and lymphatic health.

- ♥ **A question to ponder:** Can I see how much better life feels when I celebrate... compared to living in disappointment and frustration?

*The wellspring of good health
can be found
in your TOTAL lifestyle.*

*It's the wonderful gift
of living a life that works for you
on EVERY level.*

♥

Did you know that the wellspring of good health can be found in *your total lifestyle*? Oh yes! It's the ever wonderful gift of living a life that works for you on every level. And only you can do this for yourself. No one else but you!

Let's look at this together. Our lifestyle impacts our health, and living with emotional wisdom is one of the leading factors. However, there is a group of lifestyle choices, and they also include regular exercise, stress reduction, diet, cleansing, supplemental support, proper rest, sunshine, joy, water, etc.

You were born as a part of Nature, so an easy and smart thing to do for lifestyle guidance is to look at how Nature survives.

For example, take healthy wild animals. They have space to wander and be who they are. They rest when they are tired. They eat natural foods from Nature. They don't eat foods that contain antibiotics, preservatives, pesticides, etc.

Also, consider this. Animals have a similar body makeup to ours. For instance, an ape is about our size and has a comparable long intestinal tract. What do apes eat?... mostly raw fruits and greens. Why? Because it works! It helps whatever goes in to come out in a timely fashion. Likewise, in order to cleanse our long intestinal tract, we need foods that come and go easily.

Isn't it great to think of ourselves as precious beings that need consideration and care? And by thinking this way, you get to treat yourself as a precious being. So eat organic raw food with each meal. Why? There's a reason beyond it being good for your digestion. In addition, it's because this is the only food you eat that is alive and full of nutrients and vitamins – plus there's no pesticides. Cooked food, although it tastes delicious, lacks in nutrients. Any food heated above 115 degrees loses it energy. Do you get what I'm saying? Energy begets energy. That's why raw food gives you the feeling of "I could go and go and go and still feel great." And by the way... you'll look great too when you eat raw foods!

Now if you're wondering how you can make sure that you get all the nutrients you need in your diet on a daily basis, there's a company I like that has the perfect answer – *Isagenix International*. The Isagenix system is designed to be used in conjunction with daily meals. It offers you the gifts of Vitamins and Minerals, Antioxidants, plus Cleansing, Immunity Support, and Fat Burning. This is a full supplemental proven program that even offers a meal replacement shake that is enjoyable, delicious, fills you up, and cleans you out. Are you happy to find a company that gives you a full spectrum of supplements to supply what you need? You'll find more info at www.lymphforlife.isagenix.com.

The key is to stop, look and listen to your body. For instance, think about the sort of energy you have when you feel lethargic. At these times, that is exactly the kind of energy you present to yourself, others, and your lymph system. This is not a healthy state!!... the low energy, stress, and apathy – not a pretty picture! This is when you've got to get moving!! Find something you enjoy, and get yourself moving and grooving. YOU CAN DO IT!!

Yes, your nervous system and lymphatic system depend on exercise to function optimally! Daily movement that you enjoy will lift you up and relax that precious body and mind of yours. With it, you become fun, funny, adorable, attractive, and sexy.

By the way, the best form of movement for the whole body and especially the lymphatic system is rebounding – which I'll talk about more in the back pages of this book. And the Rolls Royce of Rebounders is called The Lympholine™. It's designed in a unique way and has spring-loaded legs that absorb all the impact and yet gives you a full body exercise with no jarring or trauma to the bones, skeletal system, and joints. Rebounding is aerobic, bone-building, most efficient, and LOTS OF FUN! On top of it all, it offers quick results. Learn more at the site www.lymphforlife.com.

On another note, my little two-year-old grandbaby Grace has been telling everyone, "Be quiet!" Well, from the mouth of babes come pure jewels. She's right! Make it a habit to stop, sit, close your eyes, breathe and meditate for a while each day. Get in touch with yourself and find out who you are. This will help you to follow your own lead... unlike when you go go go and never stop long enough to be in touch with yourself. YOU want to know who you are so you can be who you are. Why not?... that is the purpose of life.

Can you take it all in? *Just know that you deserve a healthy lifestyle, and so does your total being!* Without sunshine, movement, proper nourishment, and exercise, not even you want to be around yourself – let alone other people!

Well, the truth is that you are perfect! You are a gift! So you need to honor yourself by living a lifestyle that gives you the highest honors! That's why you were given life... to love, laugh, let go, honor, and obey yourself. So go, be, and enjoy this special gift called life!

Thank you for caring about yourself enough to support this precious being called YOU!

All my love,

Judy Taylor
The Lymphomaniac and a Believer in You!

♥

*We need to understand how important it is
to keep our lymphatic system healthy,
as it will enable us to live a healthier,
more energized, more joyful life...
Til the last moment.*

Mandooh Ghoneum, Ph.D.,
A Leading Expert in Cancer Immunology

♥

America's Health Needs Help!

It is apparent that America's health challenges and diseases resulting from exposure to stressful lifestyles, toxins, and the environment need to be acknowledged. The American Cancer Society (ACS) states that three-quarters of all cancer cases are the result of environmental and lifestyle factors, including air pollutants, toxins in food, lack of physical activity, etc. Today, according to the ACS, one out of every two men, and one out of every three women, are likely to develop cancer. Wow! These are statistics that will stay in our consciousness.

The condition of our lymphatic system (our internal garbage disposal system) is one of the most important factors influencing whether or not we can detoxify efficiently and feel healthy, energized and balanced.

As Mandooh Ghoneum, Ph.D., School of Medicine, University of California, Los Angeles – one of the foremost experts in cancer immunology – puts it: "The Lymphatic System is the defense system of the body. It is like the army and the intelligence agency for the country. If it is strong, the country is strong, safe and well protected. If it is weak, the country can be destroyed and occupied easily, not only from the outside, but also from the destructive enemies inside. We need to understand how important it is to keep our lymphatic system healthy, as it will enable us to live a healthier, more energized, more joyful life... Til the last moment."

In China, an ancient form of lymphatic therapy called the Art of Gua Sha is widely used as a "folk technique" in households to both prevent or treat illness. It has also long been a tool there for practitioners of Traditional Chinese Medicine. In Europe, lymphatic drainage is a very popular therapy, used for health maintenance and disease prevention. In these countries, lymphatic therapy is keeping people rejuvenated, energized, and healthy, while helping them feel and look younger. It's now time for more Americans to tap into the support that the amazing lymphatic system can provide!

You Can Lift Your Lymph!

Balance your life with factors that support the optimum functioning of your lymphatic system...

♥ The release of stress

♥ Daily fun, laughter and happiness

♥ Peaceful rest

♥ Unconditional love

♥ Movement that promotes a toned and flexible body

♥ Listening to yourself

♥ Creative expression

♥ Strong digestion

♥ Your challenges can be dealt with and are not overwhelming.

♥ Pleasant weight

♥ So called "problems" are seen as opportunities.

♥ Sexual energy is balanced.

♥ Relationships are supportive, enjoyable and supported.

♥ Your life is purposeful.

Are You Or Are You Not Congested In Your Lymphatic System?

What causes congestion?

- ♥ Stagnation (lack of movement)

- ♥ Trapped energy

- ♥ Trauma (physical or mental)

- ♥ Repressed communication

- ♥ Poor diet

- ♥ Illness

- ♥ Chemicals/drugs

- ♥ Judgment and blame

- ♥ Not listening to yourself

- ♥ Being overweight

- ♥ Rigidity

- ♥ Flabby/untoned

- ♥ Poor circulation

- ♥ Lack of exercise

- ♥ Off balance

- ♥ Overdoing

What's the result?

- ♥ Lumps, bumps, swelling in the lymphatic system

- ♥ Fatigue

- ♥ Pain

- ♥ Loss of feelings of well-being

- ♥ Disease/ill health

<u>You do</u> *with...*

- ♥ Discipline

- ♥ Movement

- ♥ Deep breathing

- ♥ Lots of water

- ♥ Organic unprocessed foods

- ♥ Truth

- ♥ Fresh air

- ♥ Relaxation

- ♥ Balance

- ♥ Self-expression

- ♥ Stress reduction

- ♥ Compassion rather than judgment and blame

- ♥ Unconditional love for yourself and others

- ♥ The LYMPHOLINE Fitness Rebounder

Lymphatic Fitness And Health That's Easy And Fun For All Ages!

There's one exercise that has more of an impact on our lymphatic health than any other form of exercise, and that is **REBOUNDING**. It consists of bouncing on a specially made mini-trampoline called a rebounder.

Remember, to keep the lymphatic fluids flowing, IT IS UP TO US TO STAY ACTIVE!

Bouncing (rebounding) specifically addresses the body's lymphatic system. Acting as the body's missing lymphatic pump, this movement activates your body's lymphatic system so it can drain away potential poisons and protect you against disease.

Better Lymphatic Health In Motion
Why The Lympholine™ Versus A Traditional Trampoline?

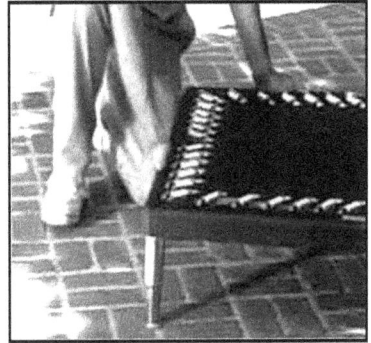

According to Lymph Specialists, the Lympholine is "The Jaguar of Rebounders"! Why was this unique piece of exercise equipment designed? Because *it supports detoxification*.

The lymphatic system is three to four times larger than the blood vessel system. It is the garbage disposal system of the inside of the body, and its fluid needs to move and flow. However it has no pump. That's why the Lympholine is a good thing.

Additional Benefits of The Lympholine™

- ♥ Unique rectangular shape will never tip over
- ♥ Ease of using increases your energy which puts it above all other trampoline/rebounders
- ♥ Lots of people get injured on other rebounders
- ♥ No injuries on the Lympholine for 12 years
- ♥ Enjoyable even if injured
- ♥ Won't get tired of using the Lympholine, compared to other rebounders
- ♥ Softest bounce

In his article "Jumping for Health," Dr. Morton Walker explains that bouncing on poorly constructed equipment (store-bought trampolines) may actually be harmful to one's muscles, joints, lymphatic system and nerves. There's no yield to them and the abrupt jarring effect is similar to landing on the floor. Ouch! You don't want that.

Just 15-30 minutes of continuous bouncing on the Lympholine provides a vigorous aerobic workout without the injuries usually associated with aerobic exercise. This leads to such benefits as lymphatic flow, toned muscles, weight loss, and increased oxygen levels, which boost immunity and result in better overall physical and mental health.

"I have tried other mini tramps, but nothing compares to the Lympholine! Cleansing of the lymphatic system, ease on the joints, and increased energy are just a few of the benefits I have experienced. I would recommend it to anyone and everyone." – T. Patton, Asheville, N.C.

The Lympholine is safety tested by one of the nation's leading testing facilities and backed by quality craftsmanship and a manufacturer's warranty. It absorbs all the harmful impact into the unit rather than your skeletal system. This alone will minimize your risk of injury while directing the equipment to maximize your health.

For more info, go to: www.lymphforlife.com.

For Kids!

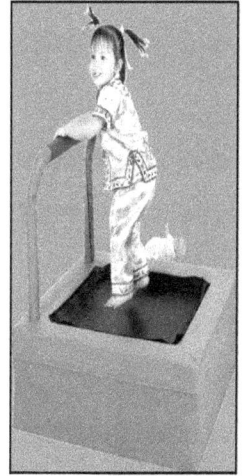

Kid's Bouncer

Did you know that one in six children in the U.S. today is overweight, triple the amount in 1980? In some areas of the country, it's even worse. In New York City, a study by the Health and Education Departments found that almost 50% of children of school age were either overweight or obese. By age three, according to the Bogalusa Heart Study, children show signs of fatty deposits in their coronary arteries. These deposits often continue to thicken through the teen years. To insure safety and greater health for our kids, get their lymphatic systems and bodies moving while they're also enjoying themselves.

The Lympholine Kid's Bouncer is a fun way to help children...

- ♥ Stay in shape and maintain appropriate body weights
- ♥ Reduce their fatty deposits and develop healthy hearts
- ♥ Provide oxygen to their blood and tissues
- ♥ Speed the correction of coordination problems

For more info, go to www.lymphforlife.com and click on "The Kid's Bouncer" box.

Read The Testimonials!

"Go Bananas in Vancouver, B.C. has installed a bouncer. It is so popular that kids are lined up to take their turn. We plan to include them in all our Toddler Playground designs that we can. It's a great play and exercise event for all toddlers."

– T. Forbes, International Play Company, British Columbia, Canada

"Gymboree Play and Music of the San Fernando Valley, in Los Angeles, has been using the Kid's Bouncer as a mainstay in our playscape of equipment for two years now. We operate the oldest Gymboree Play and Music franchise. We offer classes for parents and children newborn to 5 years old, and this piece of play equipment is extensively used daily and continues to perform as it did when it was new. The parents continually comment on its effectiveness in teaching their children about balance and also attest to the fact that it is so much fun to be able to bounce on it. The Kid's Bouncer is a fabulous piece of play equipment, engineered with great thought and expertise. I would highly recommend it in any program that is geared to young children."

– Donny Becker, Gymboree Play and Music

"We installed a bouncer in one of their locations. It is so popular that the kids are lined up to take their turn. Also they just called to ask where their 2nd one is for their new location. They plan on putting them into all their new locations. We at International play Co., plan to include them into all of our Toddler Playground Designs that we can. It's a great play and exercise event for all Toddlers."

– Terry Forbes, President, International Play Co.

The Lympholine is by far the best rebounder on the market. I personally use mine several times a week and love it. I recommend it to clients for cardiovascular and lymphatic health, and they notice the results of improved energy and and increased sense of well-being. Many pieces of exercise equipment end up stored in the garage, in the trash, or at Goodwill. This doesn't happen with the Lympholine. In addition to it's great health benefits, it is a lot of fun to use!!!

– Dr. Patricia Fitzgerald, Founder, Santa Monica Wellness Center, Author, *The Detox Solution*

"In our 2-week Living Foods LifestyleTM self-healing program, we educate students about the vital importance of maintaining healthy lymphatic systems through rebound exercise. LympholineTM is not only easy to use and gentle on the joints, but also a heck of a lot of fun! Our staff and students consider the LympholineTM to be the Rolls RoyceTM of rebounding trampolines on the market today. We really appreciate the first-class construction and ultra-smooth bounce!"

– David Williamson, Rebounding Instructor, Ann Wigmore Natural Health Institute

I received a LYMPHOLINE from my boyfriend on my 50th birthday ...and I GLADLY dumped my previous rebounder in the nearest dumpster. It was like I had been driving a 1964 Dodge Dart and traded up to a Rolls Royce! I have a friend who is a star performer in Cirque de Soleil here in Las Vegas. He came over for a visit, was "wowed" by the LYMPHOLINE and immediately started doing a routine on it. He's used to professional gymnastics equipment and was very impressed by the quality, feel and suspension system of this mini-trampoline. Personally, I use it every day, without fail, "to energize my whole body and keep my cellulite under control. As a nurse, I realize the importance of stimulating the lymphatic system, so my LYMPHOLINE is always out and accessible ...and I wouldn't ever want to be without it."

– Rosemary Duma, R.N., Las Vegas, Nevada

"I want to thank you for providing me with a LympholineTM. I have a very busy schedule and do not always get to my exercise class and now with the LympholineTM, I have the convenience of having a beneficial exercise program at home. Since I have been using the LympholineTM, I have more energy and stamina. Also, I have enjoyed the benefits of increased circulation within my body and very toned muscles."

– Laara K. Londir, Ph.D.

"I have sold and distributed the LympholineTM and Kid's Bouncer for over 4 years now, and I personally have found that my overall health and well-being had increased 100-fold with renewed energy and strength. Over the past 4 years, I have heard many good comments from my customers telling me how the LympholineTM has improved their health. There are a couple of things that seem to make the LympholineTM stand out and separates it from all other lymphatic machines on the market today. One is it size. It is 2 ½ times bigger than any other machine being sold today. Second, the springs in the legs reduces stress on joints and the skeletal system. No other machine has this. I'm very honored to be associated with Judy Taylor and the LympholineTM systems. The LympholineTM has become a part of our healthy lifestyle."

– Jim Pratt, Pratt Enterprises, Inc.

"The Lympholine rebounder, while great for exercise, is also designed to act like the missing lymphatic pump in order to support detoxification."

– Jordan S. Rubin, N.M.D., Ph.D., Author of the New York Times Bestseller, *The Maker's Diet*

The Art Of Gua Sha Kits

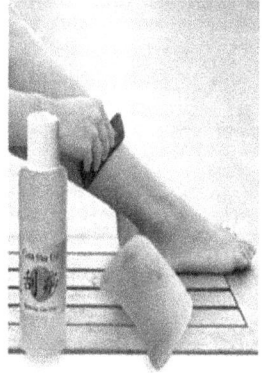

The Art of Gua Sha is a 2,000-year-old Chinese method of promoting lymph, blood and chi circulation. Its effect is achieved by stroking the skin in a particular way with a tool made of jade or water buffalo horn. This ancient technique is often used by practitioners of Traditional Chinese Medicine (TCM), but it is also a folk remedy and self-help tool widely utilized in households in China and other areas of the Far East.

Life Source International offers Gua Sha kits that include a contoured Gua Sha tool. An explanatory illustrated booklet is also enclosed. The kit with the jade tool is $133; and the one with water buffalo horn tool, $76. Discounts are available for group orders. Order a kit or request info by emailing lymphforlife@earthlink.com or calling 888-391-3719.

Acknowledgments

Every individual's life and any creative endeavor is influenced and impacted by other people. Standing in my shoes, I am forever grateful and blessed to have had the enormous influence, guidance, and support of so many.

My father was an example of openness to learning, growing, and changing, and he was brave enough to shift his life and follow his passion at sixty years old. He is my hero. My wonderful sister Susan is consistently rooting for me. My son Josh is always available with brilliant ideas, acceptance, and love, regardless of what's going on in his life. My daughter-in-law Meredith shows me that the truth will set you free and make you a better person. My grandchildren – Madison, Grace, Sean, Brianna, and Emily – opened my heart up to love in ways I never knew possible. My daughter April is always there with gentle, encouraging, and loving words. My son Michael is my example of outstanding courage. My niece Adina, my precious love, listens and encourages me along the way. My nephew David is a supportive, wonderful, caring, and dedicated man.

And to Syd Wartell, I have great gratitude for standing by me with support and love along the way.

Rachel and Barry Brooks, you are friends who have always been there on a consistent basis. My Goddess Camp sisters – Joy, Lorraine, Penny, Miriam, Shama, Beanie, Genevieve, Terri, and Jackie – you lovingly guided me back on track to complete this book and follow my passion. Judy Levy, your encouraging words, love, and belief in this project kept me moving forward on a daily basis. John Tierney, you were there at any given moment with computer support, love, and then care for my cat GiGi so I could complete this book in Sedona, Arizona. Patricia Fitzgerald, you are an example of excellence, and a constant source of support and praise. Herb Schroeder, you were always there at the drop of a pin for whatever needed to be done.

My life continues to be enriched by the many clients, students, and participants who have attended private sessions, classes, workshops, and seminars with me for the past 18 years. From all of these profound influences, I continue to be inspired to grow and become a better person.

My outstanding editor, Robin Quinn, with her editorial gifts and talents, vision, precision, attention, and competence, helped me bring the book in my mind to life. Her clarity, impeccable detail, enthusiasm, flexibility, and keen insight were invaluable.

And for my layout specialist Hillary Rogers...you made it all beautifully presented with a dedication that I will always be grateful for.

I have unlimited gratitude for all of you!

About The Author

Judy Hiney Taylor is an expert in lymphatic health. She received her training at the University of Lymphology in Utah and has been certified as a Lymphatic Specialist since 1988. In Taylor's early years as a lymphatic therapist, she saw that the lymph system was not only a wonderful physical cleanser of the body, but also an amazing detoxifier of the emotions. Taylor has been tracking the physical and emotional benefits of her work for over one and a half decades. Today she works as a Lymphatic and Emotional Release Specialist.

The author is also the Founder and CEO of Life Source International, a firm that manufactures premier rebounders for lymphatic health and fitness. Life Source International also offers the Art of Gua Sha self-help kits, used to stimulate lymph and blood circulation.

A bout with thyroid cancer was Taylor's wake-up call. After discovering the lymph/mind/health connection, she decided to devote her life to assisting others in preventing illness where possible and regaining health where necessary.

Taylor leads professional seminars for people in the lymphatic arts, other areas of healthcare, and related fields, as well as fun and educational workshops for the general public, speaking throughout the country as well as abroad.

She has appeared on numerous television and radio programs, including Fox Primetime News, educating her audiences about the importance of lymphatic health. The author teaches at the Learning Annex and has been featured in many publications.

"It is my belief that good health and peace on earth are related and they begin inside each one of us," says Taylor.

Don't forget to love yourself.

Soren Kierkegaard, Danish Philosopher and Theologian
and Judy

♥